Diagnosis and Management of Acute Otitis Media

Third Edition

Stan L. Block, MD

President, Kentucky Pediatric Research
Associate Clinical Professor of Pediatrics
University of Kentucky College of Medicine
and the University of Louisville School of Medicine

Christopher J. Harrison, MD, FAAP

Professor of Pediatrics and Pediatric Infectious Diseases
Children's Mercy Hospital and Clinics
and University of Missouri at Kansas City

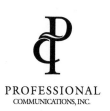

PROFESSIONAL
COMMUNICATIONS, INC.

Professional Communications, Inc.

A Medical Publishing Company

Marketing Office:
400 Center Bay Drive
West Islip, NY 11795
(t) 631/661-2852
(f) 631/661-2167

Editorial Office:
PO Box 10
Caddo, OK 74729-0010
(t) 580/367-9838
(f) 580/367-9989

For orders only, please call
1-800-337-9838

or visit our website at
www.pcibooks.com

ISBN: 1-932610-03-0

Printed in the United States of America

DISCLAIMER

The opinions expressed in this publication reflect those of the authors. However, the authors make no warranty regarding the contents of the publication. The protocols described herein are general and may not apply to a specific patient. Any product mentioned in this publication should be taken in accordance with the prescribing information provided by the manufacturer.

This text is printed on recycled paper.

DEDICATION

Stan L. Block, MD, and Christopher J. Harrison, MD, would like to dedicate this book to our wives, Melinda Block and Jane Harrison, respectively, for their patience and support throughout its writing.

ACKNOWLEDGMENT

Stan L. Block gratefully acknowledges the following mentors throughout his career: Jimmy Simon, MD, who thoroughly taught me general pediatrics; George McCracken, MD, Jerome Klein, MD, and Steve Pelton, MD, for their invaluable support and critiques of my otitis media work.

Christopher J. Harrison acknowledges Virgil Howie, MD, who taught me the art of tympanocentesis; David Welch, PhD, for setting me on the path of microbiology; D. Thomas Upchurch, MD, who gave me my first "faculty" position; and Stephen A. Chartrand for being a supportive friend when I needed it.

TABLE OF CONTENTS

TABLES

FIGURES

COLOR PLATES

1 Introduction

Otitis media (inflammation of the middle ear) accounts for a large number of outpatient visits to health care providers, and these have been on the increase: in 1975 there were 9.9 million visits to health care providers for otitis media and in 1990 there were 24.5 million visits, a rate of increase far exceeding that of population growth.[1] Furthermore, the annual cost of treating acute otitis media (AOM) in the estimated 14 million children under the age of 5 years who have this disease is more than $3 billion.[2]

As a result of its impact on health care resources, otitis media has been subjected to intense scrutiny, particularly in the past decade. Reports of a number of seminal clinical trials, meta-analyses, and clinical guideline study groups stress the importance of precision in diagnosis and management of two major types of middle ear inflammation:

- AOM
- Otitis media with effusion (OME).

Both types of inflammation are characterized by middle ear effusion (MEE).

Acute otitis media is acute infection of the middle ear as indicated by MEE, plus signs of acute inflammation. The tympanic membrane (TM) signs of acute inflammation include bulging or fullness, decreased mobility and opacification, marked erythema, or otorrhea. AOM is induced by pathogenic bacteria and/or viruses, and it is defined by the appearance of an inflamed TM and the presence of purulent MEE that usually contains pathogens. A sterile MEE (middle ear fluid without pathogens) may be present before AOM develops, and it is normal for a postinflammatory MEE to persist for weeks to months after AOM resolves.

Otitis media with effusion is a minimal inflammation of the middle ear with a nonpurulent MEE. It usually contains no pathogens or small inoculum of nonpathogenic bacteria. OME may precede, follow, or be independent of AOM.

Differentiation between AOM and OME is essential because antibiotic therapy provides a modest but significant benefit in treating AOM but is not indicated for treating OME. The critical clinical distinction between AOM and OME is the appearance of the TM.

Terms and Abbreviations

In the United States, an episode of AOM is diagnosed on the basis of TM appearance and presence of MEE. The episode ends when acute inflammatory signs resolve, regardless of the number of courses of antibiotics administered, as long as no more than 7 days elapsed between the end of one course of therapy and the start of the next.

Using these definitions, the following types of AOM may be described based on the time-course of clinical signs of infection and their response to antibiotic therapy:

- *Early-onset AOM* refers to a first episode of AOM occurring before 6 months of age.
- *Persistent AOM* refers to signs and symptoms of AOM that continue >72 hours after the start of antibiotic therapy.
- *Refractory AOM* refers to signs of AOM that persist in the week posttherapy.
- *Recurrent AOM* refers to signs with or without symptoms of AOM that recur 7 to 30 days after the last antibiotic dose.

Children are considered *otitis prone* when they have:

- Three episodes of AOM in 6 months
- Four episodes of AOM within 12 months.

Some experts also consider a child to be otitis prone after two episodes of AOM before pneumococcal conjugate vaccine (PCV)–7 within the first 6 months of life.[3] A recent study of children in rural Kentucky by the authors indicates that up to 40% of children have their first AOM by 6 months.[4]

Table 1.1 lists terms and abbreviations used in diagnosing and treating AOM.

Burden of AOM

In the United States, AOM is the most frequent diagnosis in infants and young children seen for illness visits. Most episodes of AOM can be treated effectively without permanent sequelae. However, complications of AOM can occur, including (very rarely) intracranial complications such as meningitis. Furthermore, because prolonged, repeated episodes of AOM in early childhood are accompanied by MEE that can last for weeks with transient hearing loss, AOM was thought to have a small but significant effect on language-based development.[5] Recent data suggest that prolonged effusions as long as 6 months do *not* cause measurable deficits in cognitive or language skills by school age.[6,7]

The prevalence of AOM caused by antibiotic-resistant bacteria rose dramatically in the United States during the 1990s, making treatment of AOM more difficult. The increasing risk of refractory AOM consequently may increase the risk of sequelae. Despite these difficulties, following a rational approach to diagnosing and treating AOM should have a significant positive impact on the burden of this disease on children and society. One new tool to reduce AOM is the

TABLE 1.1 — Terms and Definitions Used in Diagnosis and Treatment of Acute Otitis Media
(in alphabetical order)

Term (Abbreviation)	Definition
Acute otitis media (AOM)	Bulging or fullness, marked hyperemia, cloudy or purulent opacification of TM, or otorrhea occurring spontaneously or through a ventilating tube
Early-onset AOM	A first episode of AOM occurring before 6 months of age
Persistent AOM	Signs and symptoms of AOM that continue ≥72 hours after the start of antibiotic therapy
Refractory AOM	AOM present within 7 days posttherapy
Recurrent AOM	Signs and symptoms of AOM that recur within 7 to 30 days of the last antibiotic therapy
Antibiotic failure	Signs and symptoms of AOM that persist during therapy or after completion of a course of antibiotic therapy
Centers for Disease Control (CDC) and Prevention	Federal agency that regulates epidemiologic testing and intervention in the United States

Drug-resistant *Streptococcus pneumoniae* (DRSP)	Alternative nomenclature for PNSP
Eustachian tube (ET)	Passage between nasopharynx and middle ear
Food and Drug Administration (FDA)	In the United States, the federal regulatory agency for all pharmaceutical products and medical devices
Middle ear effusion (MEE)	Fluid in the middle ear (nonpurulent or purulent)
Moraxella catarrhalis	Third most common AOM pathogen; >95% produce β-lactamase
Nontypeable *Haemophilia influenzae* (ntHi)	In the past, ntHi was the second most common AOM pathogen; but with the routine use of pneumococcal conjugate vaccine 7, *H influenzae* accounts for 56% to 57% of pathogens in recurrent/refractory AOM, with approximately 55% to 64% producing β-lactamase in recent studies from the United States
Otitis media (OM)	Both AOM and OME
Otitis media with effusion (OME)	Inflammation of the middle ear with nonpurulent MEE
Otitis-prone child	A child who has had ≥3 episodes of AOM in 6 months or 4 episodes in 12 months

Continued

Term (Abbreviation)	Definition
Penicillin-nonsusceptible *S pneumoniae* (PNSP)	*S pneumoniae* with evidence of resistance to penicillin on susceptibility tests (such as E-test, microdilution, or broth agar) (penicillin MIC ≥0.1 µg/mL)
Intermediate-level PNSP (PNSP-I)	PNSP with penicillin MIC ≥0.1 and <2.0 µg/mL
Resistant PNSP (PNSP-R)	PNSP with penicillin MIC ≥2.0 µg/mL
Penicillin-susceptible *S pneumoniae* (PSSP)	*S pneumoniae* with penicillin MIC <0.1 µg/mL
Respiratory syncytial virus (RSV)	Respiratory virus pathogen associated with bronchitis and wheezing frequently causing secondary AOM
Rhinosinusitis	Signs similar to URI but increasing in intensity 10 days postonset, usually bacterial but frequently viral in origin
Tympanic membrane (TM)	Eardrum; 3-layered membrane separating the outer from the middle ear
Upper respiratory infection (URI)	Signs and symptoms of infection (usually viral, sometimes bacterial, rarely fungal or other) in the nasopharynx or occasionally the sinuses

PCV-7, which has some effect on AOM overall, but more specifically on the seven serotypes in the current vaccine (see Chapter 6, *Basis for Antibiotic Selection*). It may also reduce complications of pneumococcal AOM.

REFERENCES

1. Dowell SF, Marcy SM, Phillips WR, Gerber MA, Schwartz B. Otitis media—principles of judicious use of antimicrobial agents. *Pediatrics.* 1998;101(*suppl*):165-171.

2. Gates GA. Cost-effectiveness considerations in otitis media treatment. *Otolaryngol Head Neck Surg.* 1996;114:525-530.

3. Block SL. Chemoprophylaxis for the otitis-media-prone child? *Pediatric Infections Forum.* 2000;2:3, 7.

4. Block SL, Harrison CJ, Hedrick J, Tyler R, Smith A, Hedrick R. Restricted use of antibiotic prophylaxis for recurrent acute otitis media in the era of penicillin non-susceptible Streptococcus pneumoniae. *Int J Pediatr Otorhinolaryngol.* 2001;61:47-60.

5. Paradise JL, Dollaghan CA, Campbell TF, et al. Language, speech sound production, and cognition in three-year-old children in relation to otitis media in their first three years of life. *Pediatrics.* 2000;105:1119-1130.

6. Paradise JL, Feldman HM, Campbell TF, et al. Effect of early or delayed insertion of tympanostomy tubes for persistent otitis media on developmental outcomes at the age of three years. *N Engl J Med.* 2001;344:1179-1187.

7. Shriberg LD, Friel-Patti S, Flipsen P Jr, Brown RL. Otitis media, fluctuant hearing loss, and speech-language outcomes: a preliminary structural equation model. *J Speech Lang Hear Res.* 2000;43:100-120.

2 Epidemiology

Acute otitis media (AOM) is the most frequently diagnosed bacterial illness in the United States. Reported incidences may vary due to differences in study methods (failure to differentiate otitis media with effusion [OME] vs AOM, diagnostic techniques and criteria, methods for identifying cases, schedule for observations) and variations in risk factors, such as the year and season of the study and population characteristics.[1]

Incidence of AOM and Viral Upper Respiratory Infection

Epidemiologic, clinical, and laboratory studies show that viral upper respiratory infections (URIs) increase the risk for eustachian tube (ET) dysfunction and an episode of AOM. The incidence of AOM is particularly high during epidemics of URI caused by respiratory syncytial virus and influenza A.[2] (Also see Chapter 3, under the section entitled *Microbiology of Acute Otitis Media.*)

Incidence of AOM and Age

Acute otitis media is primarily a disease of young children. Between 85% and 97% of patients referred to otolaryngology clinics for insertion of tympanostomy tubes are younger than 3 years of age,[1] and most of the 28 million cases of AOM estimated to have occurred in 1993 in the United States were in children younger than 36 months.[3] Furthermore, almost all young children experience AOM; data show that in a rural Kentucky population with a 60% day care enrollment from 1989 to 1998, up to 94% of children had experienced at least one episode of AOM by age 24 months (**Figure 2.1**).[4] Prior to 1990, the incidence was lower.

Although AOM is a problem in young children worldwide, the average age at first episode and the prevalence of AOM in a given age group differ according to:

- Rates of enrollment in day care
- *Age and location.* The age at first episode of AOM differs, with more AOM at an earlier age in rural vs urban populations (**Figure 2.1** and **Figure 2.2**).
- *Age and time period.* Comparison of incidence by age for earlier and more recent time periods in the United States shows that children in the 1990s experienced their first episode of AOM at a younger age than in the past (**Table 2.1**).
- *Age and type of AOM.* First episode of AOM occurring at a younger age is a strong predictor both of persistent middle ear effusion (MEE), refractory AOM, and recurrent AOM[5]

The demographics of the 1970s urban vs the 1990s rural population were remarkably similar (smoking, breast-feeding, indigent population, siblings, race), except for the rate of day care, which was negligible in the Boston group and ranged from 50% to 65% in rural Kentucky (**Figure 2.2**). Day care appears to be the major factor associated with increased rates of AOM being observed in the 1990s. In populations with high rates of day care, not only do more children experience AOM, but they also experience nearly 2-fold more episodes of AOM annually.

Although most episodes of AOM occur in children younger than 3 years who have a preceding or concurrent viral URI, not all young children with URIs

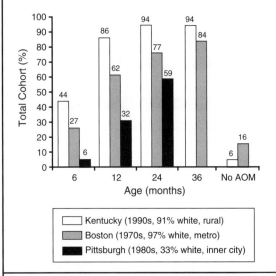

FIGURE 2.1 — Cumulative Percentage of Children With First Episode of Acute Otitis Media in Three Populations

Teele DW, et al. *J Infect Dis.* 1989;160:84-94; Casselbrant ML, et al. *Int J Pediatr Otorhinolaryngol.* 1995;33:1-16; Block S, et al. *Int J Pediatr Otorhinolaryngol.* 2001;61:47-60.

develop AOM. Therefore, other risk factors must contribute to the incidence of AOM. **Table 2.2** lists risk factors for AOM according to whether they are inherent (not modifiable, likely to be related to the patient's anatomy and physiology) or environmental (potentially modifiable, except for season).

Inherent Risk Factors

Inherent risk factors for AOM include:
- Genetic factors
- Environmental factors (exposures during fetal development).

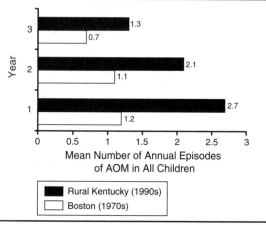

FIGURE 2.2 — Mean Annual Rate of Episodes of Acute Otitis Media in First 3 Years: Boston vs Rural Kentucky

Abbreviation: AOM, acute otitis media.

Rates of day care were unreported but believed to be minimal in the Boston group and ranged from 55% to 60% in the rural Kentucky group.

Data from: Teele DW, et al. *J Infect Dis.* 1989;160:84-94 and Block SL, et al. *Int J Pediatr Otorhinolaryngol.* 2001;61:47-60.

TABLE 2.1 — Worldwide Cumulative Incidence of Acute Otitis Media by Age

Age (y)	Cumulative % With at Least One Episode of Acute Otitis Media
1	15 to 62
2	35 to 71
3	46 to 84

Summarized from statistics reported by Casselbrant ML, Mandel EM. Epidemiology. In: Rosenfeld RM, Bluestone CD, eds. *Evidence-Based Otitis Media.* St. Louis, Mo: BC Decker; 1999:117-137.

TABLE 2.2 — Risk Factors for Acute Otitis Media

Inherent Risk Factors

- Age <24 months
- Male gender
- Down syndrome
- Midface abnormalities
  - Cleft palate
  - Choanal atresia
- Family history of frequent acute otitis media
- Frequent acute otitis media or history of pressure-equalizing tubes
- Maternal smoking during pregnancy
- Ethnicity:
  - Native Alaskan
  - Native American
  - White race
- Immunologic problems
  - Antibody deficiencies (Bruton's agammaglobulinemia, IgG2 subclass deficiency,[1] poor polysaccharide antigen antibody responders)

Environmental Risk Factors

- Upper respiratory tract infection
- Season of the year (fall through spring)
- Bottle-feeding rather than breast-feeding
- Pacifier use
- Siblings in household
- Smoking in household
- Day care/group care (>5 attendees)
- Managed-care health insurance coverage
- Lower socioeconomic group
- Lack of being fully vaccinated with the pneumococcal conjugate vaccine (PCV)–7

[1]Veenhoven R, et al. *Pediatr Res.* 2004;55:159-162.

■ **Genetic Factors**

Genotype

A recent prospective study in monozygotic or dizygotic twin and triplet sets found that the number of episodes of AOM correlates closely with genetic heritage, independent of gender and other risk factors such as socioeconomic status.[6] According to the investigators, this finding suggests that genetics play a large role in MEE. Genetically related factors (inherited anatomic and immunologic) shown to be related to increased risk of AOM include:

- Greater pneumatization of the mastoid process
- A shorter, straighter eustachian tube (such as is found in Native Americans and Down syndrome children)
- Human leukocyte antigen (HLA)-A2 and not HLA-A3 in children with recurrent AOM
- Presence of the IgG2 genetic marker G2m(23) in children with recurrent AOM.

Male Gender

In some studies, there was a significantly higher incidence of AOM and more episodes of recurrent AOM in males than in females, and males have also been reported to be more prone to persistent MEE.[1]

Midface Abnormality/Down Syndrome

The incidence of AOM and OME is significantly higher in children with unrepaired cleft palate, craniofacial abnormality, and Down syndrome, probably due to the effects of abnormal anatomy, such as softer cartilage and narrower caliber, on ET function.[1,7]

Maternal Smoking in Pregnancy

Stathis and colleagues found that the number of cigarettes the mother smokes during pregnancy is directly correlated with the risk of middle ear disease during the first 5 years of life.[8] Likewise, Lieu and Feinstein showed that continued passive smoke exposure after maternal gestational smoking further increases risk of recurrent AOM.[9]

2

White Race

In their review of several studies in the United States, Casselbrant and Mandel found that white children have a higher incidence of AOM and middle ear abnormalities compared with African-American children.[1] In addition, comparison of results in two prospective studies conducted in major metropolitan areas in the northeastern United States in the 1970s, one with a mostly white study group[5] in the 1990s and one with a study group that was only 33% white,[10] indicates earlier onset of first episode of AOM in the predominantly white study group (**Figure 2.1**).

In confirmation of these findings, the incidence of AOM is also higher in white compared with African-American children in one author's (SB) population in rural Kentucky. A recent study shows that in a nonurban area with a high rate of day care, the risk for recurrent AOM in white vs African-American children is 3.7-fold and 13.7-fold higher in year 1 and year 2, respectively (**Figure 2.3**).

In contrast, a study of inner-city African-American and white children that sought to control for all other risk factors, such as socioeconomic background, found no significant difference by race in incidence of otitis media (OM) (when both AOM and OME were included) in children followed monthly and examined when symptoms occurred during the first 2 years of life.[10] However, the rates at which children were enrolled in day care were not reported.

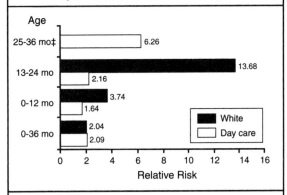

FIGURE 2.3 — Major Relative Risk for Recurrent Acute Otitis Media (or Otitis-Prone Condition*)†

* See *Terms and Abbreviations* in Chapter 1, *Introduction* for the definition of otitis prone.
† All patients; by multivariate analysis with $P < 0.05$.
‡ No increase listed for white children.

Data from: Block SL, et al. *Int J Pediatr Otorhinolaryngol.* 2001;61:47-60.

Native Americans

Studies show a higher incidence of recurrent episodes of OM, chronic MEE, and chronic suppurative OM in some Native American populations both in the continental United States and Alaska. This increased incidence of AOM has been linked to the results of comparative anatomic studies that show that many Native American populations have shorter, straighter ETs.[11,12]

■ Environmental Risk Factors

Environmental risk factors for AOM include exposures to upper respiratory tract pathogens, factors that affect immune system function, and factors that affect access to health care.

Season

Viral URIs, OME, and AOM are diagnosed more frequently in the northern hemisphere during the fall and winter seasons and least often in the summer. On the other hand, the prevalence of drug-resistant *Streptococcus pneumoniae* has been found to be higher in late winter and spring.[13]

Bottle-Feeding vs Breast-Feeding

Breast-feeding exclusively for 4 months or longer has been associated with significantly fewer episodes of AOM, and prolonged breast-feeding (6 months or longer) has been reported to offer even greater protection, according to a review of studies by Casselbrant and Mandel.[1] Sassen and colleagues found that the full protective effects of breast-feeding last 4 months after breast-feeding is discontinued and disappear 12 months after discontinuation.[14] Casselbrant and Mandel suggested that the benefits of breast-feeding could be:

- Immunologic factors:
  - Antibodies against respiratory tract viruses and bacteria
  - Factors that prevent bacterial adhesion
  - Avoidance of allergens in formulas
- Mechanical factors:
  - Better development of facial muscles that support ET function
  - Less chance of aspiration of fluids into the middle ear
  - Feeding position that discourages reflux.

Sibling in Household

In the United States, a study of AOM in white and African-American children from the same socioeconomic background followed monthly to age 2 years found that both African-American and white infants who were firstborn had less ear disease (episodes of AOM and MEE) than those who had older siblings.[10] Similarly, other studies have found that children with more siblings are more likely to have recurrent AOM.[7,15]

Day Care

The findings of numerous studies[15-19] indicate that one of the most significant factors in the increasing burden of AOM is the trend toward almost universal enrollment, for at least some period of time, of preschool-age children in day care. In fact, children in day care with at least five other children have at least twice the risk of developing AOM compared with children cared for at home.[16] In addition, day care is an important risk factor for early-onset AOM and refractory or drug-resistant AOM.[4] Block and associates showed a twofold greater risk for recurrent AOM among rural children in day care during the first 3 years of life.[4]

A family history of atopy adds to the risk that a child in day care will have URI and AOM. Among a group of children with a family history of atopy who were followed during their first year of life, those who attended day care were found to have 3.2 times the incidence of rhinorrhea as those in home care and 2.4 times the risk of two or more episodes of AOM. They also had a higher incidence of sinusitis (2.2 times) and a higher incidence of lower respiratory tract infection (1.6 times).[18]

Pacifier Use

Children younger than 3 years in day care who use pacifiers are at increased risk for AOM.[19] Limited use of pacifiers among children under 24 months may decrease the rate of AOM by 30%.

Enrollment in Managed Care Plan and Lower Socioeconomic Status

Less access to health care, which has been thought to be associated with enrollment in a managed care plan or lower socioeconomic status, has been postulated to reduce the incidence of diagnosed AOM. If one looks at the presence of MEE due to OME or AOM, one study found an inverse relationship between days with MEE and socioeconomic status; but many studies showed no correlation between socioeconomic status and incidence of MEE.[1] However, in these studies, a majority of days with MEE were due to OME, not AOM. Therefore, the increased risk of AOM with higher socioeconomic status may predict more frequently diagnosed AOM. Some differences may be related to rates of day care enrollment.

Role of Pneumococcal Conjugate Vaccine

Poehling and colleagues studied the population impact of pneumococcal conjugate vaccine (PCV)–7 on pneumococcal-related diseases.[20] They examined two US populations before (1995–2000 in Tennessee; 1998–2000 in New York) and after (2000–2002) PCV-7 licensure. They observed an overall reduction in the rate of AOM resulting from PCV-7 vaccination (6% in Tennessee and 20% in upstate New York). Additionally, they found that the ratios of otitis media visits to the emergency department and in the outpatient setting declined by 16% and 4%, respectively, in Tennessee, and declined by 41% and 19%, respectively, in New York.[20]

REFERENCES

1. Casselbrant ML, Mandel EM. Epidemiology. In: Rosenfeld RM, Bluestone CD, eds. *Evidence-Based Otitis Media*. St. Louis, Mo: BC Decker; 1999:117-137.

2. Ruuskanen O, Arola M, Putto-Laurila A, et al. Acute otitis media and respiratory virus infections. *Pediatr Infect Dis J.* 1989;8:94-99.

3. US Department of Health and Human Services. *Vital and Health Statistics. Current Estimates from the National Health Interview Survey, 1993.* Hyattsville, Md: Public Health Service, Centers for Disease Control and Prevention, National Center for Health Statistics; 1994.

4. Block SL, Harrison CJ, Hedrick J, Tyler R, Smith A, Hedrick R. Restricted use of antibiotic prophylaxis for recurrent acute otitis media in the era of penicillin non-susceptible Streptococcus pneumoniae. *Int J Pediatr Otorhinolaryngol.* 2001;61:47-60.

5. Teele DW, Klein JO, Rosner B. Epidemiology of otitis media during the first seven years of life in children in greater Boston: a prospective, cohort study. *J Infect Dis.* 1989; 160:83-94.

6. Casselbrant ML, Mandel EM, Fall PA, et al. The heritability of otitis media: a twin and triplet study. *JAMA.* 1999;282: 2125-2130.

7. Saenz RB. Primary care of infants and young children with Down syndrome. *Am Fam Physician.* 1999;59:381-396.

8. Stathis SL, O'Callaghan DM, Williams GM, et al. Maternal cigarette smoking during pregnancy is an independent predictor for symptoms of middle ear disease at five years' postdelivery. *Pediatrics.* 1999;104:e16.

9. Lieu JE, Feinstein AR. Effect of gestational and passive smoke exposure on air infections in children. *Arch Pediatr Adolesc Med.* 2002;156:147-154.

10. Casselbrant ML, Mandel EM, Kurs-Lasky M, Rockette HE, Bluestone CD. Otitis media in a population of black American and white American infants, 0-2 years of age. *Int J Pediatr Otorhinolaryngol.* 1995;33:1-16.

11. Doyle WJ. A functional-anatomic description of Eustachian tube vector relations in four ethnic populations: an osteologic study [PhD dissertation]. Pittsburgh, Pa: University of Pittsburgh, 1977.

12. Beery QC, Doyle WJ, Cantekin EI, Bluestone CD, Wiet RJ. Eustachian tube function in an American Indian population. *Ann Otol Rhinol Laryngol.* 1980;89(suppl):28-33.

13. Boken DJ, Chartrand SA, Goering RV, et al. Colonization with penicillin-resistant *Streptococcus pneumoniae* in a child-care center. *Pediatr Infect Dis J.* 1995;14:879-884.

14. Sassen ML, Brand R, Grote JJ. Breast-feeding and acute otitis media. *Am J Otolaryngol.* 1994;15:351-357.

15. Kero P, Piekkala P. Factors affecting the occurrence of acute otitis media during the first year of life. *Acta Paediatr Scand.* 1987;76:618-623.

16. Kvaerner KJ, Nafstad P, Hagen J, Mair IW, Jaakkola JJ. Early acute otitis media: determined by exposure to respiratory pathogens. *Acta Otolaryngol Suppl.* 1997;529:14-18.

17. Sipila M, Karma P, Pukander J, Timonen M, Kataja M. The Bayesian approach to the evaluation of risk factors in acute and recurrent acute otitis media. *Acta Otolaryngol.* 1988; 106:94-101.

18. Celedon JC, Litonjua AA, Weiss ST, Gold DR. Day care attendance in the first year of life and illnesses of the upper and lower respiratory tract in children with a familial history of atopy. *Pediatrics.* 1999;104:495-500.

19. Niemela M, Uhari M, Mottonen M. A pacifier increases the risk of recurrent acute otitis media in children in day care centers. *Pediatrics.* 1995;96:884-888.

20. Poehling KA, Lafleur BJ, Szilagyi PG, et al. Population-based impact of pneumococcal conjugate vaccine in young children. *Pediatrics.* 2004;114:755-761.

3 Pathophysiology, Immunology, and Natural History

The pathophysiology of acute otitis media (AOM) primarily involves eustachian tube (ET) dysfunction, which is influenced by anatomic, genetic, and immune system factors.

Anatomy of the Eustachian Tube

The anatomy of the ET changes with age. From infancy to the ET's maturity when the child is about age 7 years, the ET lengthens, cartilage increases in amount, firmness, and density, and the angle of the ET to the horizontal plane changes from about 10° (allowing easy reflux of materials in the nasopharynx) to about 45°.[1]

A number of anatomic factors in addition to immaturity can affect ET function, including:

- Anatomic abnormalities present from birth (such as cleft palate or deviated nasal septum)
- Injury, neoplasm, or surgery involving structures in or near the ET complex, such as the nose, palate, pterygoid bone, tensor veli palatini muscle, mandibular branch of the trigeminal nerve, and nasopharynx.

Function of the Eustachian Tube

The ET, which connects the nasopharynx to the middle ear space, functions in concert with the nasopharynx, nose, soft and hard palates, middle ear, and mastoid air cells to:

- Regulate pressure in the middle ear (ventilatory function) — a normally functioning ET equalizes pressure in the middle ear to the atmospheric pressure
- Protect the middle ear (protective function) from sound-pressure changes and reflux of secretions from the nasopharynx to the middle ear
- Clear secretions produced in the middle ear (clearance function) into the nasopharynx.[1]

Functions of the ET system are shown schematically in **Figure 3.1**.

Mechanisms of Eustachian Tube Dysfunction

Anatomic and pathologic factors that can impair ET function include:
- Inflammation (acute or chronic) of tubal mucosa or surrounding tissues
- A polyp or cholesteatoma near the tube lumen
- Compression of the tube by a tumor or adenoid mass
- A shorter tube (promotes reflux of secretions)
- A "floppy tube" (inefficient action of muscles to open the tube)
- Tubal stenosis (rare).

All infants and young children have impaired ET function due to immature anatomy of the tube. Virtually all infants and young children with cleft palate have severe impairment of ET function.[1]

The mechanisms that can affect ET function include:
- Excessive negative middle ear pressure (such as occurs when taking off in an airplane)

FIGURE 3.1 — Functions of the Eustachian Tube System

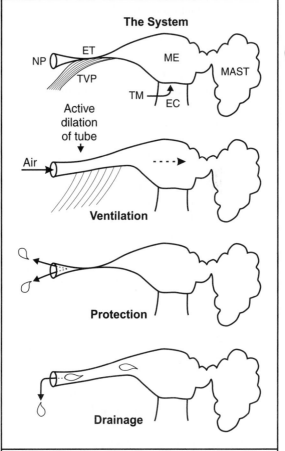

Abbreviations: EC, external canal; ET, eustachian tube; MAST, mastoid air cells, ME, middle ear, NP, nasopharynx; TM, tympanic membrane; TVP, tensor veli palatini muscle.

Bluestone CD. *Pediatr Infect Dis J.* 1996;15:281-291.

- Excessive positive nasopharyngeal pressure (nose-blowing, forceful crying, or descent in an airplane)
- Negative nasopharyngeal pressure (sucking on a bottle or pacifier or swallowing), which, if the ET is patent, can lead to negative middle ear pressure (the Toynbee phenomenon)
- Rapid change in ambient pressure (such as occurs during ascent or descent in an airplane or underwater diving)
- Exposure to cigarette smoke
- Loss of middle ear gas cushion (perforation of tympanic membrane or radical mastoidectomy)
- Impaired function of cilia (likely in those with a genetically inherited ciliary dysmotility disorder or after repeated infection/injury secondary to bacteria, viruses, or irradiation)
- Ineffective tubal pumping action due to negative pressure in the middle ear
- Impaired mastoid cell pneumatization[2] occurs genetically in some children but is also induced by AOM episodes at a young age or frequent intervals. Poor mastoid pneumatization provides less reserve for middle ear pressure maintenance so that lesser pressure fluctuations result in more rapid depletion of oxygen content of the middle ear. This in turn increases the drive for goblet cell replication and mucous production. Placement of pressure-equalizing (PE) tubes prevents oxygen depletion and normalizes goblet cell numbers and function.
- Excessive goblet cell numbers also can occur due to AOM without changes in pneumatization. Cytokines in middle ear fluid appear to stimulate replication of goblet cells. More goblet cells cause more mucous production that peaks 8 to 16 days after the AOM episode.[3] This mucus is more acidic than the usually neutral pH. Both

increased mucous volume plus lower pH add to persistence of middle ear effusion (MEE). Nontypeable *Haemophilus influenzae* (ntHi) induces more mucous than the other AOM pathogens. This may explain why ntHi is the most frequent isolate in MEE of otitis media with effusion (OME) (up to 12%).

- Pneumococcus, more than ntHi or *Moraxella catarrhalis*, induces middle ear mucosal cell enzyme activity (cysteine proteases), which increases the severity of mucosal injury and accompanying ET dysfunction.

Microbiology of AOM

The pathogenesis of AOM involves local immune system changes in response to viruses, allergens, and bacterial pathogens.

The major bacterial pathogens in AOM are *Streptococcus pneumoniae*, *H influenzae*, *M catarrhalis*, and group A *Streptococcus*. Factors affecting the relative incidence of AOM caused by these pathogens are discussed at length in Chapter 6, *Basis for Antibiotic Selection*.

■ Viruses

A meta-analysis by Ramilo of nine studies involving 1024 children conducted from 1982 to 1996 found:

- Viruses were detected in an average 19% (range 8% to 25%) of MEEs obtained by tympanocentesis after AOM was diagnosed according to strict criteria
- A virus was the sole pathogen isolated in only about 5% of cases.[4]

Heikkinen and colleagues also report finding only a viral pathogen in about 6% of cases of AOM.[5] They studied viruses in the pathogenesis of AOM in a group of 456 children and were able to identify a specific virus in the nasopharynx causing the concurrent upper respiratory infection (URI) in 186 children (41%). They were able to isolate virus from the MEE in 77 of these 186 cases. Not only did respiratory syncytial virus (RSV) cause the majority of cases of URI, it was the most likely pathogen to be found in MEE of AOM (**Table 3.1**).

Another study reported the prevalence of viruses and bacteria in nasopharynx secretions and/or MEE of children 3 months to 7 years of age with AOM, using culture and polymerase chain reaction (PCR):

- Virus was detected in 62% of nasopharyngeal samples and in 48% of MEEs
- Bacterial pathogens were detected in 62% of MEEs
- Viral nucleic acids were detected in 57% of MEEs without bacteria and in 45% of those with bacteria.[6]

Recent data indicate that up to 17% of children hospitalized with RSV have accompanying AOM.[7] In a Scandinavian study later than that of Heikkinen and colleagues, RSV was not confirmed as the predominant viral pathogen during accompanying AOM, being only 10% vs 38% for rhinovirus and 23% for enteroviruses.[8] This likely represents the natural cyclic nature of viral disease from season to season.

In summary, viral URI is usually the initial step in the development of AOM. But isolation of virus by culture as the sole pathogen in AOM occurs in only 5% to 6% of cases.

■ Allergens and the Inflammatory Response in AOM

Allergens affecting the nasopharynx have long been suggested as a cause of altered ET function and thus a risk factor for AOM. In addition to respiratory

TABLE 3.1 — Viruses in the Upper Respiratory Tract and Middle Ear Effusion in 186 Children With Acute Otitis Media

Virus	URTIs Caused by Virus (n = 186)	MEEs Containing Virus (n = 77)
Respiratory syncytial virus	65 (35%)	48/65 (74%)
Parainfluenza viruses	29 (16%)	15/29 (52%)
Influenza viruses	24 (13%)	10/24 (42%)
Enteroviruses	27 (15%)	3/27 (11%)
Adenoviruses	23 (12%)	1/23 (4%)

Abbreviations: MEE, middle ear effusion; URTI, upper respiratory tract infection.

Heikkinen T, et al. *N Engl J Med.* 1999;340:260-264.

allergy, some clinicians believe that IgG-mediated food allergy is important in the development of recurrent MEE in young children.[9] However, no current allergy therapy has been convincingly shown to reduce AOM frequency.

■ Bacteria in AOM

Although viruses are frequent triggers and occasional pathogens for AOM, *bacteria are the major pathogens of AOM.* The primary role of viral pathogens in the etiology of AOM is in provoking the initial inflammatory response. Viruses have been found to be the sole pathogens in only about 5% to 6% of cases of AOM,[3] but in most other cases, bacteria (either alone or with viruses) are responsible for the signs and symptoms of AOM. Three studies have shown that bacterial pathogens can be isolated in 87% to 95% of cases by using optimal culture methods.[10,11] A majority of sterile MEEs from AOM where no bacteria are isolated are likely due to bacteria that were killed by the host immune system, suboptimal culture technique, or surreptitious or intentional previous antibiotic use.

■ Summary of the Pathogenesis of AOM

The pathogenesis of AOM is summarized in **Figure 3.2**.[12]

Time-Course and Possible Outcomes of AOM

In a study of 421 episodes of AOM in 352 children attending day care (mean age 2.1 years), Heikkinen found that the onset of symptoms of AOM occurred most often on the third day after the onset of symptoms of viral infection.[12,13]

Dowell and colleagues analyzed studies of the duration of MEE after resolution of AOM and found that MEE can last for 1 to 3 months in 60% of children

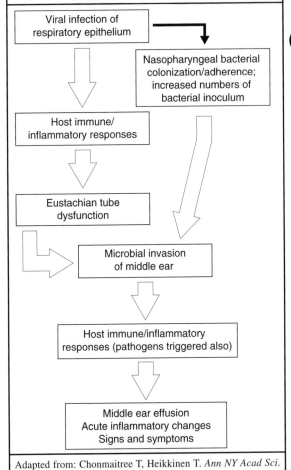

FIGURE 3.2 — Pathogenesis of Acute Otitis Media After Respiratory Viral Infection

Viral infection of respiratory epithelium

Nasopharyngeal bacterial colonization/adherence; increased numbers of bacterial inoculum

Host immune/inflammatory responses

Eustachian tube dysfunction

Microbial invasion of middle ear

Host immune/inflammatory responses (pathogens triggered also)

Middle ear effusion
Acute inflammatory changes
Signs and symptoms

Adapted from: Chonmaitree T, Heikkinen T. *Ann NY Acad Sci.* 1997;830:149.

after pathogens have presumptively been eradicated from the middle ear.[14]

Figure 3.3 diagrams the typical time course of AOM after upper respiratory tract infection and the possible outcomes of AOM diagnosed on day 0.

Studies[15,16] indicate that in patients who undergo tympanocentesis, their AOM will be resolved without an effective antibiotic:

- In about 20% of cases of *S pneumoniae* infection
- In about 50% of cases of AOM caused by *H influenzae*
- In 50% to 80% of cases of AOM due to *M catarrhalis*.

REFERENCES

1. Bluestone CD. Pathogenesis of otitis media: role of eustachian tube. *Pediatr Infect Dis J.* 1996;15:281-291.

2. Valtonen HJ, Dietz A, Qvarnberg YH, Nuutinen J. Development of mastoid air cell system in children treated with ventilation tubes for early-onset otitis media: a prospective radiographic 5-year follow-up study. *Laryngoscope.* 2005;115:268-273.

3. Caye-Thomasen P, Tos M. Eustachian tube gland changes in acute otitis media. *Otol Neurotol.* 2004;25:14-18.

4. Ramilo O. Role of respiratory viruses in acute otitis media: implications for management. *Pediatr Infect Dis J.* 1999; 18:1125-1129.

5. Heikkinen T, Thint M, Chonmaitree T. Prevalence of various respiratory viruses in the middle ear during acute otitis media. *N Engl J Med.* 1999;340:260-264.

6. Pitkaranta A, Virolainen A, Jero J, Arruda E, Hayden FG. Detection of rhinovirus, respiratory syncytial virus, and coronavirus infections in acute otitis media by reverse transcriptase polymerase chain reaction. *Pediatrics.* 1998; 102:291-295.

7. Kafetzis DA, Astra H, Tsolia M, Liapi G, Mathioudakis J, Kallergi K. Otitis and respiratory distress episodes following a respiratory syncytial virus infection. *Clin Microbiol Infect.* 2003;9:1006-1010.

8. Nokso-Koivisto J, Raty R, Blomqvist S, et al. Presence of specific viruses in the middle ear fluids and respiratory secretions of young children with acute otitis media. *J Med Virol.* 2004;72:241-248.

9. Bernstein JM. Role of allergy in eustachian tube blockage and otitis media with effusion: a review. *Otolaryngol Head Neck Surg.* 1996;114:562-568.

10. Block SL, Harrison CJ, Hedrick, JA, et al. Penicillin-resistant *Streptococcus pneumoniae* in acute otitis media: risk factors, susceptibility patterns and antimicrobial management. *Pediatr Infect Dis J.* 1995;14:751-759.

11. Rodriguez WJ, Schwartz RH. *Streptococcus pneumoniae* causes otitis media with higher fever and more redness of tympanic membranes than *Haemophilus influenzae* or *Moraxella catarrhalis*. *Pediatr Infect Dis J.* 1999;18:942-944.

12. Heikkinen T. Role of viruses in the pathogenesis of acute otitis media. *Pediatr Infect Dis J.* 2000;19(suppl 5):S17-S23.

13. Heikkinen T. Temporal development of acute otitis media during upper respiratory tract infection. *Pediatr Infect Dis J.* 1994;13:659-661.

14. Dowell SF, Marcy SM, Phillips WR, Gerber MA, Schwartz B. Otitis media—principles of judicious use of antimicrobial agents. *Pediatrics.* 1998;101(suppl):165-171.

15. Howie VM, Ploussard J, Sloyer JL, Hill JC. Use of pneumococcal polysaccharide vaccine in preventing otitis media in infants: different results between racial groups. *Pediatrics.* 1984;73:79-81.

16. Marchant CD, Carlin SA, Johnson CE, Shurin PA. Measuring the comparative efficacy of antibacterial agents for acute otitis media: the 'Pollyanna phenomenon'. *J Pediatr.* 1992;120:72-77.

FIGURE 3.3 — Possible Outcomes of Acute Otitis Media

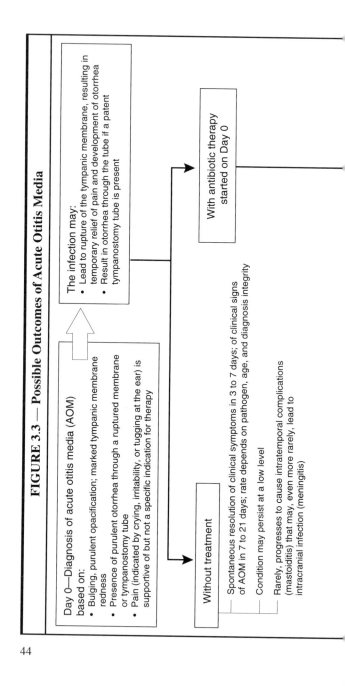

Day 0—Diagnosis of acute otitis media (AOM) based on:
- Bulging, purulent opacification; marked tympanic membrane redness
- Presence of purulent otorrhea through a ruptured membrane or tympanostomy tube
- Pain (indicated by crying, irritability, or tugging at the ear) is supportive of but not a specific indication for therapy

The infection may:
- Lead to rupture of the tympanic membrane, resulting in temporary relief of pain and development of otorrhea
- Result in otorrhea through the tube if a patent tympanostomy tube is present

Without treatment
- Spontaneous resolution of clinical symptoms in 3 to 7 days; of clinical signs of AOM in 7 to 21 days; rate depends on pathogen, age, and diagnosis integrity
- Condition may persist at a low level
- Rarely, progresses to cause intratemporal complications (mastoiditis) that may, even more rarely, lead to intracranial infection (meningitis)

With antibiotic therapy started on Day 0

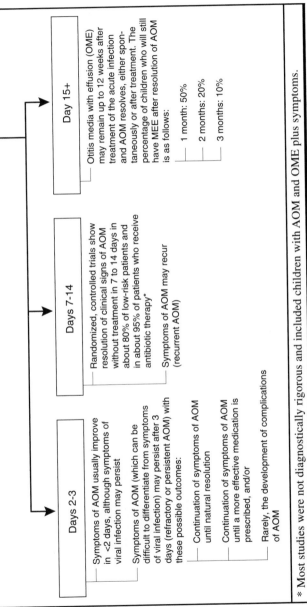

Days 2-3

Symptoms of AOM usually improve in <2 days, although symptoms of viral infection may persist

Symptoms of AOM (which can be difficult to differentiate from symptoms of viral infection) may persist after 3 days (refractory or persistent AOM) with these possible outcomes:

- Continuation of symptoms of AOM until natural resolution

- Continuation of symptoms of AOM until a more effective medication is prescribed, and/or

- Rarely, the development of complications of AOM

Days 7-14

Randomized, controlled trials show resolution of clinical signs of AOM without treatment in 7 to 14 days in about 80% of low-risk patients and in about 95% of patients who receive antibiotic therapy*

Symptoms of AOM may recur (recurrent AOM)

Day 15+

Otitis media with effusion (OME) may remain up to 12 weeks after treatment of the acute infection and AOM resolves, either spontaneously or after treatment. The percentage of children who will still have MEE after resolution of AOM is as follows:

- 1 month: 50%

- 2 months: 20%

- 3 months: 10%

* Most studies were not diagnostically rigorous and included children with AOM and OME plus symptoms.

3

4 Diagnosis

Symptoms alone are insufficient to diagnose acute otitis media (AOM) and practitioners should not rely on parental history for the diagnosis. Supporting symptoms, such as fever and otalgia, are present in AOM only in 25% of younger children and in 50% of older ones. Furthermore, symptoms are not necessary to support the diagnosis of AOM, which is a visual diagnosis that should be based upon the following two elements:

- Objective documentation of the presence of middle ear effusion (MEE)
- Visual signs of middle ear inflammation and/or purulence by pneumatic otoscopy.

The diagnosis of AOM can only be made when the visual findings of or behind the tympanic membrane (TM) correlate with the presence of pus (or leukocytes) or marked hyperemia, which usually indicates the presence of bacteria.[1-3] These criteria are similar to other diagnostic criteria for bacterial infection in any other body site. For instance, the presumptive diagnosis of pneumonia cannot be based solely upon the presence of cough, tachypnea, or fever, but rather requires the presence of rales, absent breath sounds, or radiographic infiltrate. Fortunately, the TM provides a window to the middle ear cavity to discern whether pus or noninflammatory MEE or merely air is present behind the TM.

The lack of viable bacteria detectable by culture from a purulent MEE (no growth in 5% to 30% of cases) does not negate the diagnosis of AOM. This is similar to the scenario when pus (pleocytosis) but no bacterial growth occurs in the cerebrospinal fluid, which also does not negate the diagnosis of meningitis.

AAP/AAFP Guideline

The 2004 American Academy of Pediatrics and the American Academy of Family Physicians (AAP/AAFP) guideline[4] requires the presence of *each of the following three elements* before a diagnosis of AOM can be "certain" (**Table 4.1**):

1. Abrupt onset of signs and symptoms of middle-ear inflammation
2. Presence of middle ear effusion (MEE) indicated by:
   • Bulging TM
   • Reduced TM mobility
   • Air-fluid level
   • Otorrhea
3. Signs or symptoms of TM inflammation, including:
   • Distinctly reddened TM
   • Otalgia.

The guideline does not clearly give a definition of what factors must constitute the elements of "abrupt onset." Some experts state that there must be documented abrupt onset of Criteria 2 (MEE) and Criteria 3 (signs and symptoms of TM inflammation) before a diagnosis of AOM is "certain." However, a clinician cannot document elements of either otorrhea or otalgia as being of "abrupt onset" unless the child has been examined recently. The clinician will rarely be able to document the acute onset of bulging of the TM, reduced TM mobility, air-fluid level, or distinct redness of the TM. Thus without the presence of an abrupt onset of otorrhea or otalgia, a distinctly reddened TM or bulging pus-filled TM will always be relegated to the

TABLE 4.1 — Definition of AOM According to AAP/AAFP 2004 Guideline

A diagnosis of AOM requires:
- A history of acute onset of signs and symptoms
- The presence of MEE, and
- Signs and symptoms of middle ear inflammation

Elements of the definition of AOM are all of the following:
- Recent, usually abrupt, onset of signs and symptoms of middle ear inflammation and MEE
- The presence of MEE that is indicated by any of the following:
  - Bulging of the TM
  - Limited or absent mobility of the TM
  - Air-fluid level behind the TM
  - Otorrhea
- Signs or symptoms of middle ear inflammation as indicated by either:
  - Distinct erythema of the TM or
  - Distinct otalgia (discomfort clearly referable to the ear[s] that results in interference with or precludes normal activity or sleep)

Abbreviations: AAP, American Academy of Pediatrics; AAFP, American Academy of Family Physicians; AOM, acute otitis media; MEE, middle ear effusion; TM, tympanic membrane

AAP/AAFP. *Pediatrics*. 2004;113:1451-1465.

category of uncertainty or otitis media with effusion (OME) per the current guideline.

Other experts think that the text on this matter (as stated in the first sentence of the guideline) infers that "fever, otorrhea, irritability, and otalgia" might be the signs and symptoms that are the categories necessary for "abrupt onset." However, the guideline contradicts such thoughts because it also clearly states that clinical history is poorly predictive of AOM and such signs and symptoms are nonspecific.

For instance, fever, "earache," or excessive crying was present not only in 90.1% of patients with AOM but also in 72.4% of patients without AOM.[5] Furthermore, only 67.7% of children <2 years of age with AOM had any ear-related symptoms.[5] Niemela and colleagues concluded that AOM does not consistently cause symptoms that parents can use in their decision to seek medical attention for their child.

The authors of the guideline declared that the best study evaluating middle ear findings that correlate with AOM are derived from the Karma study.[6,7] However, two caveats must be noted with this study. First, the investigators performed myringotomy without culture. While symptoms needed to be present in order to diagnose AOM, the symptoms they used were wide ranging and often very nonspecific (eg, fever, earache, irritability, ear rubbing or tugging, other simultaneous acute respiratory symptoms, vomiting, or diarrhea[7]).

Nonetheless, this study may be the most thorough one ever performed on MEE attempting to differentiate symptomatic AOM from nonsymptomatic MEE. It involved 5,462 children with acute symptoms and MEE, and 1,092 children with MEE but no acute symptoms. But even in this study, espoused by the authors of the Guideline as the benchmark for AOM, TM redness showed poor sensitivity for the diagnosis of AOM. TM redness was seen in only 21% of children who had AOM (defined as acute symptoms with MEE present). TM redness was predictive of MEE in only half of the children with AOM. As such, a red TM was "an inconsistent finding . . . an unreliable indicator in AOM." Even more important, TM redness with hypomobility was a "rather rare finding with MEE" (**Table 4.2**). Thus it appears that TM redness was *not* present in nearly 80% of children with AOM in this study, and it can be present in the absence of AOM even when reduced mobility is also present.

On the other hand, in the Karma study, TM cloudiness (dullness, opacification) showed high sensitivity, specificity, and predictive value for AOM. TM bulging was also very reliably predictive of MEE and was present in one half of cases of AOM. Furthermore, impaired mobility is highly dependent on the otoscopist's skill. Even when impaired mobility may not have been present in the middle ears in this study (without cloudiness or bulging), it had low predictive value for AOM.

Our Perspective on AAP/AAFP Diagnostic Criteria

According to the AAP/AAFP guideline, a certain diagnosis of AOM must meet each of the three criteria: rapid onset, presence of MEE, and presence of signs and symptoms of middle ear inflammation. Therefore, according to the AAP/AAFP guideline, in the absence of any of the three criteria, AOM should not be the diagnosis. Rather the child would default to either the "uncertain" diagnosis or to OME (**Color Plate 1**). For example, if the TMs of the children in **Color Plate 1**, Photos A and B (retracted TMs, so definitely not AOM cases) showed reduced mobility and they presented with "otalgia or irritability," then these children would be considered to have AOM. An additional problem is that assessment of mobility is quite subjective and highly dependent on the child's cooperation, adequate instrumentation, and sufficient speculum seal. Diagnostic criteria for AOM are often inconsistent; for example, the AAP/AAFP criteria do not require the presence of a purulent MEE nor a bulging TM in order to make a diagnosis of AOM. Pneumatic portion of otoscopy is difficult, and clinicians may become so preoccupied with this part of the examination that the key components of an acutely in-

TABLE 4.2 — Middle Ear Effusion in Visits With Different Tympanic Membrane Findings (Predictive Value)

| Tympanic Membrane Finding | Middle Ear Effusion Present in Visits | | | |
| | With Acute Symptoms | | Without Acute Symptoms | |
	Group 1 (%)	Group 2 (%)	Group 1 (%)	Group 2 (%)
Color				
Red	59.6	51.4	24.0	23.0
Distinctly red*	69.8	65.6	29.5	39.3
Hemorrhagic	81.3	62.9	100.0	40.0
Strongly red	87.7	68.1	27.2	54.5
Moderately red	59.8	66.0	28.1	30.0
Slightly red	39.4	16.7	16.1	3.8
Cloudy	95.7	80.0	95.1	52.3
Normal	1.7	4.9	1.0	4.5

Position				
Bulging	96.0	89.0	95.7	81.4
Retracted	46.8	49.6	41.9	38.6
Normal	32.1	22.2	14.8	9.4
Mobility				
Impaired	86.0	68.1	79.0	40.8
Distinctly	94.0	78.5	91.5	55.8
Slightly	59.7	32.8	54.0	12.0
Normal	2.7	4.8	0.5	1.8

* Hemorrhagic, strongly, or moderately red

Karma PH, et al. *Int J Pediatr Otorhinolaryngol.* 1989;17:37-49.

flamed or purulent TM may be overlooked, as seems to be suggested by the AAP/AAFP guideline.

In contrast, in **Color Plate 1**, Photos D, E, and F, the TMs lack distinct redness. Without concurrent otalgia, according to the guideline, the lack of TM redness precludes an AOM diagnosis because these TM appearances cannot fulfill Criteria 3. More important with regard to the guideline, up to 80% of children with AOM have a bulging/full TM that is not reddened.[7] On the other hand, using the guideline criteria, any child with "otalgia" whose TM does not move or who has an air-fluid level (even if it is clearly nonpurulent) can now be considered to have AOM.

We also are concerned that the symptom of "otalgia" has been given equal diagnostic weight as a physical finding — a distinctively reddened TM in Criteria 3. We think that TM inflammation can only be defined by physical findings—either redness and opacity of the TM or the yellow-colored opaque pus behind the TM. We are concerned about the notion that symptoms must be present to define a physical diagnosis of AOM. We believe that the diagnosis of AOM should be based on visual findings and should not require nonspecific symptoms to be present to fulfill two of three elements of the guidelines.

■ **Post–Antibiotic AOM**

Within 1 week post–antibiotic therapy, children will frequently have persistent MEE with minimal or no symptoms. Yet those children who undergo tympanocentesis will frequently still have pus and bacteria detected by culture.[1,8-10] They likely have not had enough time for development of symptoms because of a sometimes slow return to rapid bacterial replication after antibiotic therapy or bacterial suppression.

■ Adjunctive Tools

The AAP/AAFP guideline states that the presence of MEE can be adjunctively established by either tympanometry or acoustic reflectometry. Yet neither instrument is designed to or capable of differentiating AOM from OME.[11] This recommendation now allows a child who has a positive instrument test and who has symptoms of recent-onset otalgia, etc, to be diagnosed as having AOM if a retracted TM is erythematous.

4

Diagnosis of AOM — Our Perspective

AOM should be defined by the presence of either purulent MEE behind a full to bulging TM or a bulging TM with marked redness and opacification. Either criterion plus bulging or fullness of the TM should almost always assure the presence of pus and usually bacteria. Among children with bona fide AOM, 87% to 95% of those with a purulent MEE will grow a typical aerobic bacteria (*Streptococcus pneumoniae, Haemophilus influenzae, Moraxella catarrhalis*, group A streptococcus).[1-3] Virus as a sole pathogen in AOM is found in only 6% of cases.[12,13]

Critical elements that clinicians should document in their examination of the TM include:

- TM position (full/bulging, neutral, or retracted): full/bulging = AOM
- Discoloration of the TM/MEE (gray, reddened, amber/orange, or purulent [gray/green, yellow, creamy white]): purulent MEE = AOM
- Translucency vs opacity of the TM (bony landmarks seen clearly or not): opacified with redness or pus = AOM
- Mobility of the TM, when possible (**Table 4.3**). It is rare not to be able to document mobility if the correct tools are used, the child is adequately restrained, and cerumen has been cleared from the canal.

55

TABLE 4.3 — Mobility of the Tympanic Membrane
• Position: A full/bulging TM = AOM • Acute otorrhea = AOM • Opacified full to bulging TM that is distinctively, markedly reddened = AOM • Opacified full to bulging TM that has a green, yellow, or creamy white purulent MEE = AOM
Abbreviations: AOM, acute otitis media; TM, tympanic membrane.

TMs that appear to have merely a pink or amber (orangish) discoloration do not indicate AOM, regardless of lack of mobility.

Symptoms of AOM

Symptoms of otalgia and fever are often associated with AOM. However, irritability in a preverbal child does not necessarily indicate otalgia, and even when pain seems to be localized to the ear region, it may be due to another condition, such as otitis externa or referred pain from tonsillar or pharyngeal pain fibers.[14,15] The nonspecific symptom of fever accompanies AOM in as few as 23% of all cases.[16] Fever is too frequently a result of the viral pathogen, and even when present with other indicators, it is an unreliable indicator for AOM. It is also an unreliable symptom upon which to conclude that an antibiotic has failed even though AOM is severe because in most cases fever is usually a result of the viral coinfection.

Despite the fact that no symptoms are sufficiently diagnostic by themselves, the presence of AOM from certain other AOM-related symptoms can be helpful in parental decision-making about the appropriateness of seeking an office visit. It is important to note the relative risk for an AOM diagnosis when different symptoms are present.

Predicting AOM Based on Symptoms of Upper Respiratory Infection

A study of symptoms of upper respiratory infection in children in day care found that the following symptoms were *associated* with AOM[17]:

- Earache
- Sore throat
- Night restlessness
- Fever, peak association from day 3 to day 9 of symptoms.

In this study, the presence of both earache and night restlessness correctly predicted the diagnosis of AOM in 71% of cases, and parents were able to predict the presence of AOM from symptoms with a sensitivity of 71% and a specificity of 80%. However, 15% of children had earache but not AOM and 41% of children with AOM did not have ear-related symptoms, confirming that ear pain is not diagnostic of AOM. In distinct contrast to the Karma study, there was no association in this study between AOM and gastrointestinal symptoms, cough, poor appetite, or rhinitis.[17]

Predicting Causative Organism Based on Symptoms

Nearly all cases of AOM in children with identified pathogens are caused by *S pneumoniae*, *H influenzae*, *M catarrhalis*, or *Streptococcus pyogenes*. Antibiotic susceptibilities of these organisms differ and tympanocentesis is rarely feasible to help choose the appropriate drug. One study evaluated whether clinical symptoms differed according to the pathogen causing AOM. There were no significant differences by pathogen in degree of pain, but significantly more febrile AOM cases (temperature of 37.8°C or higher) were due to *S pneumoniae* (40 of 65 patients [62%]) compared with *H influenzae* (20%) or *M catarrhalis* (18%). Cases of AOM with higher severity of TM redness and bulging[2] also were more likely due to *S pneumoniae* (61%) compared with *H influenzae* (25%) or *M catarrhalis* (14%). *S pneumoniae* was 4-fold more common than gram-negative β-lactamase–positive organisms among children who had severe otalgia or fever. So clinicians should target *S pneumoniae* in children who have higher fever or more severe otalgia. This is in contradistinction to the AAP/AAFP guideline, which espouses β-lactamase–positive organisms as the primary target in this highly febrile or severe otalgia scenario by virtue of a recommendation for amoxicillin plus a β-lactamase inhibitor (clavulanate) instead of amoxicillin alone when high fever is present.

Pneumatic Otoscopy

To give reliable results, pneumatic otoscopy needs to be performed with appropriate equipment (**Table 4.4**) and proper technique (**Figure 4.1** and **Figure 4.2**).

To examine most children 4 to 30 months old, the original speculum with an aperture of 3.0 mm that is 35 mm (1.375 inches) long and tapered should be used. Most children ≤4 months old require the 2.5-mm speculum. Welch-Allyn disposable specula are too dull, too narrow, too short, and inadequately tapered (**Figure 4.3**). Original specula should be cleaned with alcohol wipes, etc, after each use. However, the Otrec disposable specula from Medical Disposables Laboratories Inc. (361 Haynes Road, Dyersburg, Tenn. 38024 USA; 901-286-4211) are manufactured in full-

TABLE 4.4 — Equipment for Pneumatic Otoscopy

Item	Qualifications	Supplies/Maintenance
Pneumatic otoscope (Figure 4.2)	Must have bright halogen light source	Halogen bulbs (replace bulb when light is dull even though the battery is fresh)
	May be wall mounted or handheld	Batteries for handheld model; recharge at least daily
Specula (Figure 4.3)	Variety of sizes needed (2.5-, 3-, and 4-mm apertures) Must seal well with otoscope head Must transmit light fully to the tip Must be full-length, tapered Original equipment is best	Alcohol wipes to clean
Wire-loop cerumen curette*	Flexible loop reduces potential canal damage; stainless steel more efficient than plastic	Alcohol wipes to clean

* Wire-loop curette available from Storz Instruments, 600 Corporate Point, Culver City, CA 90230 USA (800-421-0837).

FIGURE 4.1 — Steps in Performing and Interpreting Results of Pneumatic Otoscopy

Step 1: Calm patient if necessary

⇨ Procedure will be performed at multiple visits in the first 2 years of life. Minimizing discomfort provides results most quickly, for current as well as future examinations.

Step 2: Position and restrain patient

⇨ Children are usually more at ease in the caregiver's lap. Infants may be wrapped securely in a blanket with arms at sides. Young children may lie or sit in the caregiver's lap with the inner arm snug between the child's body and the caregiver's chest; the caregiver holds the other upper arm securely against the child's side.

Step 3: Examine the canal

⇨ Rule out external canal infection or foreign body.

Step 4: Remove cerum to see tympanic membrane (TM)

⇨ Diagnosis is not reliable without viewing the entire TM. The first sign of acute otitis media (AOM), eg, fullness, may appear in the upper quadrants (pars flaccida) while perforations are often in lower quadrants.

Step 5: Assessment of TM

➡ Normal middle ear:
  - Visible landmarks
  - Neutral TM position
  - Gray to translucent

Otitis media with effusion (OME):
  - Landmarks too prominent
  - Retracted or neutral position
  - None to mild increase in TM vascularity
  - Translucent to opaque

AOM is indicated by TM:
  - Tympanostomy tube: fluid drainage—clear or purulent?
  - Otorrhea: through a tube or ruptured TM? (Purulent drainage is pathognomonic)
  - TM position: bulging or full indicates increased middle ear pressure; loss of landmarks
  - Nature of fluid behind TM: purulent effusion
  - TM translucency/opacity: white, yellow, or pale-green discoloration and opacification
  - TM color: erythema or significant injection

Continued

4

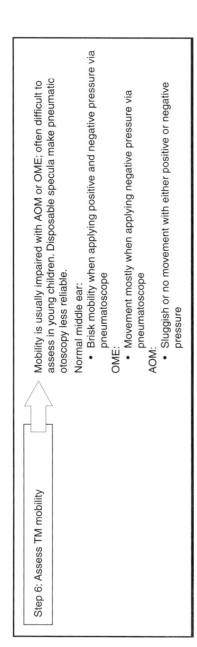

Step 6: Assess TM mobility

Mobility is usually impaired with AOM or OME; often difficult to assess in young children. Disposable specula make pneumatic otoscopy less reliable.

Normal middle ear:
- Brisk mobility when applying positive and negative pressure via pneumatoscope

OME:
- Movement mostly when applying negative pressure via pneumatoscope

AOM:
- Sluggish or no movement with either positive or negative pressure

FIGURE 4.2 — Otoscope Head and Sof-Spec Speculums

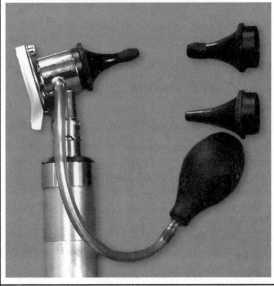

The Paradise diagnostic-head, fiberoptic, pneumatic oto-scope *(left)* has a stainless steel, barrel-shaped head with a round lens that seals via a metal clip. Bulb is attached to tubing, which in turn attaches to external metal nipple. This lens clip plus external nipple design provides longer service life for the head. Fixed specula also provide a more securely closed system compared with the twist-on–type specula required by square, plastic, TV-screen–shaped alternative otoscope head (**Figure 4.3**). Note difference in standard speculum *(just above bulb)* compared with tapered tips on Sof-Spec specula *(attached to oto-scope and in upper right corner)*. A different head with small mobile lens is preferred for use when performing tympanocentesis.

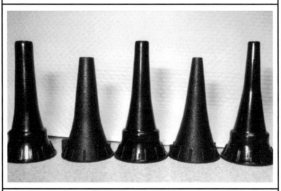

From left to right: 4.0 mm original equipment (OE) speculum, 4.0 mm disposable speculum, 3.0 mm OE speculum, 2.5 mm (actual 2.0 mm) disposable speculum, 2.5 mm OE speculum. The length of each OE speculum is $1^7/_{16}$ inch, and each disposable speculum is $1^1/_4$ inch.

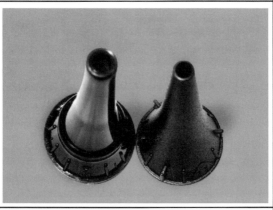

Overhead view of a 2.5 mm original equipment speculum *(left)* vs a 2.5 mm (actual 2.0 mm) disposable speculum *(right)*.

COLOR PLATE 1 — AOM, OME,
Normal, or Uncertain?

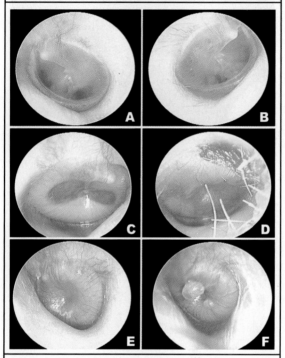

Abbreviations: AOM, acute otitis media; OME, otitis media with effusion; TM, tympanic membrane.

(A) Normal TM; (B) normal TM; (C) early purulent AOM, neutral position; (D) AOM bulging without redness; (E) bulging AOM with pus but minimal hyperemic injection; and, (F) bulging AOM with pus but minimal hyperemic injection.

Photos courtesy of David McCormick, MD, Galveston, Tex.

COLOR PLATE 2 — CDT™ Aspirator

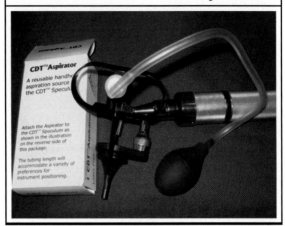

length sizes with apertures of 2.5, 3.0, and 4.0 mm, and may be adequate. When first acquiring the skill of pneumatic otoscopy, use of the nondisposable Sof-Spek (**Figure 4.2**) provides an easier seal that is less uncomfortable for the patient due to the soft tapered tips.

■ Lighting

Clinicians should use nickel-cadmium rechargeable batteries for their otoscopes. These usually require replacement about every 2 years, or they can use wall-mounted otoscopic battery packs. These also will need routine replacement once the light source becomes dim over several years. Alkaline batteries produce a meager light source in comparison and should not be used in otoscopes. Also, halogen light bulbs must be changed routinely about every 6 months or so with regular use.

Common Diagnostic Pitfalls

Avoid these pitfalls in the diagnosis of AOM:
- Mistaking the pink or light red blush from crying for TM inflammation
- Mistaking the orange/amber appearance of the TM in OME for AOM
- Assuming that presence of any TM abnormality indicates AOM
- Assuming that any air-fluid levels indicate active infection
- Assuming that decreased TM mobility alone indicates AOM
- Mistaking increased vascularity after recovery from AOM as a sign of ongoing infection
- Failing to remove occluding cerumen; about two thirds of infants <10 months old have cerumen obscuring TM visualization.

Although AOM is the most common bacterial infection seen by practicing general pediatricians, less than three lectures on AOM are delivered annually throughout their pediatric residency. When Steinbach and colleagues examined the correlation between the clinical diagnostic examination of children with AOM comparing pediatric residents with pediatric otolaryngologists, there was only slight to moderate correlation in diagnostic accuracy of the residents.[18] Steinbach and associates said that "otitis media is the most common disease seen by practicing general pediatricians, but there is a paucity of formalized resident education." The correlation between pediatric residents and pediatric otolaryngologists was only about 30% for clinical findings of the TM in 103 patients.

Pichichero and associates presented lectures on the clinical appearance of a wide variation of TM conditions. Most TM photographs consisted of OME with a few photographs of AOM or normal TMs. When participants were tested on the diagnosis, only 50% of pediatricians and 73% of otolaryngologists were able to correctly diagnose the TM appearance according to these experts.[19,20]

Otoscopic examination is imperative. AOM should not be diagnosed and treated merely on the basis of a child's history or an adjunctive instrument. This practice will lead to overprescribing of antibiotics, which exposes the child to the risk of adverse drug effects, fosters the development of antibiotic-resistant strains in the child's nasopharynx, and exacerbates the growing worldwide problem of antibiotic-resistant infections. AOM diagnosis based on history must be confirmed by otoscopy (**Figure 4.1**).

■ Can Ancillary Instruments Be Used to Diagnose AOM in Symptomatic Children?

The only technique short of myringotomy or tympanocentesis for confirming the diagnosis of AOM is pneumatic otoscopy. To confirm mobility and the likelihood of effusion, tympanometry or acoustic reflectometry can be useful. When validated against pneumatic otoscopy, both instruments showed approximately two thirds sensitivity for MEE and were about 90% accurate for absence of MEE.[11,21] Neither instrument can differentiate AOM from OME.

Tympanometry measures sound absorption at different pressures, so when the MEE occupies more of the middle ear space, less sound is absorbed, yielding a "B" curve whether the MEE is a sterile secretion or purulent material.

Both the acoustic reflectometer and the tympanometer are intended to supplement pneumatic otoscopy in defining the presence or absence of MEE. Neither is capable of differentiating AOM from OME.[21] In clinical testing,[11] the spectral gradient acoustic reflectometer accurately determined the presence of MEE in only 80% of cases, and only if the ear canal was <50% occluded with cerumen. Conversely, 15% and 20% of cases of tympanocentesis-proved AOM had a normal reading with tympanometry and acoustic reflectometry, respectively. Thus using an abnormal result from either instrument to fulfill the criteria for the presence of MEE, coupled with the presence of symptoms, will lead to many false diagnoses of AOM when OME or a normal TM is present. Conversely, a normal test result could dissuade an uncertain clinical diagnosis from an AOM diagnosis that is genuine.

REFERENCES

1. Block SL, Harrison CJ, Hedrick JA, et al. Penicillin-resistant *Streptococcus pneumoniae* in acute otitis media: risk factors, susceptibility patterns and antimicrobial management. *Pediatr Infect Dis J.* 1995;14:751-759.

2. Rodriguez WJ, Schwartz RH. *Streptococcus pneumoniae* causes otitis media with higher fever and more redness of tympanic membranes than *Haemophilus influenzae* or *Moraxella catarrhalis. Pediatr Infect Dis J.* 1999;18:942-944.

3. Del Beccaro MA, Mendelman PM, Inglis AF, et al. Bacteriology of acute otitis media: a new perspective. *J Pediatr.* 1992;120:81-84.

4. American Academy of Pediatrics Subcommittee on Management of Acute Otitis Media. Diagnosis and management of acute otitis media. *Pediatrics.* 2004;113:1451-1465.

5. Niemela M, Uhari M, Jounio-Ervasti K, Luotonen J, Alho OP, Vierimaa E. Lack of specific symptomatology in children with acute otitis media. *Pediatr Infect Dis J.* 1994;13:765-768.

6. Lieberthal AS, Ganiats TG. The overlooked importance of tympanic membrane bulging: in reply. *Pediatrics.* 2005;115: 513-514.

7. Karma PH, Penttila MA, Sipila MM, Kataja MJ. Otoscopic diagnosis of middle ear effusion in acute and non-acute otitis media. I. The value of different otoscopic findings. *Int J Pediatr Otorhinolaryngol.* 1989;17:37-49.

8. Block SL, Hedrick JA, Tyler RD, Smith RA, Harrison CJ. Microbiology of acute otitis media recently treated with aminopenicillins. *Pediatr Infect Dis J.* 2001;20: 1017-1021.

9. Casey JR, Pichichero ME. Changes in frequency and pathogens causing acute otitis media in 1995-2003. *Pediatr Infect Dis J.* 2004;23:824-828.

10. Block SL, Busman TA, Paris MM, Bukofzer S. Comparison of five-day cefdinir treatment with ten-day low dose amoxicillin/clavulanate treatment for acute otitis media. *Pediatr Infect Dis J.* 2004;23:834-838.

11. Block SL, Pichichero ME, McLinn S, Aronovitz G, Kimball S. Spectral gradient acoustic reflectometry: detection of middle ear effusion in suppurative acute otitis media. *Pediatr Infect Dis J.* 1999;18:741-744.

12. Heikkinen T. Role of viruses in the pathogenesis of acute otitis media. *Pediatr Infect Dis J.* 2000;19(5 suppl):S17-S22; discussion S22-S23.

13. Chonmaitree T. Viral and bacterial interaction in acute otitis media. *Pediatr Infect Dis J.* 2000;19(5 suppl):S24-S30.

14. Heikkinen T, Ruuskanen O. Signs and symptoms predicting acute otitis media. *Arch Pediatr Adolesc Med.* 1995;149:26-29.

15. Howie VM, Schwartz RH. Acute otitis media. One year in general pediatric practice. *Am J Dis Child.* 1983;137:155-158.

16. Block SL. Management of acute otitis media in the 1990s: the decade of resistant pneumococcus. *Paediatr Drugs.* 1999;1:31-50.

17. Kontiokari T, Koivunen P, Niemela M, Pokka T, Uhari M. Symptoms of acute otitis media. *Pediatr Infect Dis J.* 1998;17:676-679.

18. Steinbach WJ, Sectish TC, Benjamin DK Jr, Chang KW, Messner AH. Pediatric residents' clinical diagnostic accuracy of otitis media. *Pediatrics.* 2002;109:993-998.

19. Pichichero ME. Diagnostic accuracy, tympanocentesis training performance, and antibiotic selection by pediatric residents in management of otitis media. *Pediatrics.* 2002;110:1064-1070.

20. Pichichero ME, Poole MD. Assessing diagnostic accuracy and tympanocentesis skills in the management of otitis media. *Arch Pediatr Adolesc Med.* 2001;155:1137-1142.

4

21. Block SL, Mandel E, McLinn S, et al. Spectral gradient acoustic reflectometry for the detection of middle ear effusion by pediatricians and parents. *Pediatr Infect Dis J*. 1998;17:560-564; discussion 580.

5 Tympanocentesis

With the correct equipment and an experienced clinician, tympanocentesis (inserting a needle through the tympanic membrane [TM] and aspirating fluid from the middle ear) is a simple procedure that allows for:

- Immediate relief of severe otalgia
- Culture of pathogen of the middle ear effusion (MEE), particularly in refractory acute otitis media (AOM) unresponsive to multiple antibiotics
- Targeted antibiotic therapy for AOM[1]
- A pathogen to target in a toxic child with concurrent bacteremia or pneumonia.

Rationale for Tympanocentesis

The American Academy of Pediatrics and the American Academy of Family Physicians (AAP/AAFP) guideline for the diagnosis and management of AOM states that after the child fails a 3-day regimen of ceftriaxone, then tympanocentesis is recommended (**Table 7.2** and **Table 7.3**).[2]

Although tympanocentesis was the standard treatment for relief of pain from AOM in the preantibiotic era, it seemed an unnecessary procedure in the decades when antibiotic treatment yielded almost universal resolution of AOM signs and symptoms. For cases of AOM refractory to antibiotic therapy, however, the combination of tympanocentesis and culture and susceptibility testing of the pathogen in MEE is the only way to accurately select an antibiotic to which the causative pathogen is known to be susceptible.

Over the past 15 years, clinicians noted an alarming increase in the proportion of cases of AOM that did not respond to traditional antibiotic therapy. As a result, tympanocentesis was recently recommended for clinicians treating children with refractory AOM by the Drug-Resistant *Streptococcus pneumoniae* Therapeutic Working Group of the Centers for Disease Control and Prevention[3] and the 2004 AAP/AAFP guidelines.[2] Clinicians should develop the capacity to perform tympanocentesis or establish a referral network for the procedure.[3] In addition, the AAP now advocates that pediatricians perform tympanocentesis as an adjunct to manage refractory AOM (after the third antibiotic has failed to lead to clinical cure).[2] Having said that, there seems to be less refractory AOM since the onset of the universal use of pneumococcal conjugate vaccine in infants.

Table 5.1 shows advantages of tympanocentesis for refractory AOM compared with other therapies such as myringotomy with insertion of tympanostomy tubes or empiric choice of another antibiotic.

Procedure for Tympanocentesis

Tympanocentesis can be performed in the office with the assistance of a nurse and with the equipment listed in **Table 5.2**. Most practices will already have much of the equipment listed except for the collection systems.

■ Office Tympanocentesis: Step by Step

When performed by an experienced practitioner, tympanocentesis requires approximately 15 minutes of the pediatrician's time and 10 to 30 minutes of intermittent nursing time. The most time-consuming aspect is the 30 to 40 minutes required for the tetracaine anesthesia to "take." The extra time to perform this procedure is no more burdensome than the time needed to manage similar urgent conditions that are a routine occurrence in the pediatric office or clinic (ie, lacera-

Benefit/Risk	Tympanocentesis	M & T	Additional AB
Pain relief	Within 15 minutes	For M&T, 1+ week lead time to schedule	1-2 days will often suppress symptoms
Organism recovery (identification and susceptibility testing)	Up to 87% pathogen recovery rate; culture results in 1 to 3 days	Concomitant, allows for culture and susceptibility testing (but rarely obtained)	No culture
Complication risk	Serious complications extremely rare	For M&T, general anesthesia risk	Moderate likelihood of continuing infection
Time to perform	About 10 to 45 minutes (<30 seconds for actual puncture)	For M&T, time to refer to otolaryngologist	1 minute to prescribe plus follow-up and phone calls/ office visits if not effective
Patient charges	~$250 (Table 5.2); CPT codes 69420/.50 + 99142	$1500-$3000	$40-$100, depending on antibiotic choice

TABLE 5.1 — Benefits/Risks of Tympanocentesis vs Other Therapies for Refractory Acute Otitis Media

Abbreviations: AB, antibiotic (chosen without knowledge of pathogen's antibiotic susceptibility); CPT, current procedural terminology; M&T, myringotomy with insertion of tympanostomy tube.

Data from: Block SL. *Contemporary Pediatrics.* 1999;16:103-127.

TABLE 5.2 — Equipment for Office Tympanocentesis

Item	Approximate Cost	Comments
Incubator and culture plates	$300 incubator; 75¢ to $1 ea/culture plates	5% sheep blood agar and chocolate agar plates
Child restraint, such as papoose board	$300	—
Pulse oximeter with pediatric probe	$600	Only if sedation is used
Surgical otoscope head or Hotchkiss otoscope	$122/$280	Welch-Allyn or San Franciso Medical
Suction tubes, #3 and #5 Fr Baron, 7-cm metal, with thumb plate and bypass hole	$35 each	—
ONE of the following collection systems:		
1. *Alden-Senturia trap (suction dependent)*		
18-Gauge, 2.5-inch spinal needle	$3	Bend tip at 30° to 45° angle
Suction machine (to 150-200 cm H_2O)	$200-$300	Usually available in treatment room/crash cart
2-inch tubing from suction machine to trap	$6-$10	—
Alden-Senturia trap, sterilizeable	$110	Easy to use, clean in autoclave, reusable

2. *Tymp-Tap* (suction dependent)		
18-Gauge, 2.5-inch spinal needle	$3	Bend tip at 30° to 45° angle
Suction machine (to 150–200 cm H_2O)	$200–$300	—
2-foot tubing from suction machine to trap	$1/foot	—
Tymp-Tap	$150/box of 10	Easy to use, disposable
3. *Tuberculin syringe* (suction-independent)	$1	Very cumbersome; requires significant dexterity
18-Gauge, 2.5-inch spinal needle	$3	Bend tip at 30° to 45° angle
4. *Oto-Scan Laser-Assisted Myringotomy system* (suction-independent)		
Oto-LAM device	$73,000	Very easy to use, clearly shows site of incision; collection of specimen difficult, must swab tympanic membrane; perforation remains open 2 to 4 weeks; difficult to culture

Continued

5

Item	Approximate Cost	Comments
Medications:		
Nonbacteriostatic saline	$2/5-mL vial	—
Isopropyl alcohol	$1/pint	—
Topical tetracaine 8% (>80% effective)	$10-$16/patient	Compounded by pharmacist, anesthetizes in 15-30 minutes; also available in kits that do not require pharmacy compounding
Optional sedation (for patients >5 months) (drug for emergency reversal of sedation):		
Midazolam (Versed); sedative/anxiolytic agent	$402/118 mL	Dosage 0.5 to 0.7 mL, max. 20 mg/kg
Flumazenil (Romazicon); reversed agent	$36/5-mL vial	Dosage 10 μg/kg IV q 30-60 sec to max 1 mg
Resuscitation equipment (if sedation is used):		
Bag, mask, oxygen	—	Should already be available in all offices
Intravenous catheters, tubing, fluids, vasopressors	—	Should already be available in all offices
Adapted from: Block SL. *Contemporary Pediatrics.* 1999;16:103-127.		

tion, nasal foreign body). With current indications for tympanocentesis (severe/painful AOM or AOM refractory to multiple antibiotic therapy), the procedure may be needed in about 1% of office visits for AOM.

Figure 5.1 shows the step-by-step procedure for office tympanocentesis using the options of oral midazolam for sedation and/or 8% tetracaine and an Otowick for topical TM anesthesia. In the past 5 years, our practice (SLB) has opted almost exclusively for the use of topical tetracaine anesthesia without sedation.

Practitioners may want to select the easier to use Alden-Senturia collection trap or Tym-Tap hooked up to wall suction for specimen collection rather than the Tuberculin-syringe plunged with the thumb technique. The newest instrument is the CDT™ Aspirator (**Color Plate 2**), which uses a bulb syringe to aspirate. We are concerned that having the needle guided strictly by the lower end of the speculum could create a problem when entering the inferior anterior space of the TM. Also the suction generated by a bulb syringe will be insufficient for more tenacious MEE present in most refractory AOM.

In the child with severe AOM in one ear and milder AOM (eg, a purulent air-fluid level) in the other, it is useful to perform tympanocentesis on both ears because milder AOM will otherwise likely progress to severe, painful AOM.

■ **Culture Procedure**

Prepare the culture as soon as possible after aspirating MEE by:

- Carefully unscrewing the collection trap (if not using the tuberculin syringe).
- Using a sterile swab (preferred) or tuberculin syringe with needle to inoculate solid agar plates with aspirate.

FIGURE 5.1 — Steps for Performing Tympanocentesis in the Pediatric Office

Step 1: Inform family, obtain consent

1. Explain procedure to the family, including the risks and benefits
2. Review informed-consent document and obtain signatures of parents, and also patients when ≥7 years old

Step 2: Administer topical anesthetic,* consider sedative; begin monitoring if sedative used

1. Instill 8% tetracaine (3 to 5 drops) into the external canal, insert a polyester Otowick and saturate it with additional tetracaine; it will take 30-40 minutes for tetracaine to anesthetize.

NOTE: Following step should be taken only in the event that sedation is used in conjunction with topical anesthetic:

2. Administer midazolam syrup† (children >5 months only):
   a. Begin continuous pulse oximeter monitoring
   b. Nurse starts checking vital signs every 5 to 10 minutes
   c. Check for adequate sedation

Step 3: Prepare for tympanocentesis (25 to 30 minutes after topical anesthetic/administration of sedative)

1. Sterilize the external canal(s):
   a. Restrain the child
   b. If tetracaine is not used, instill isopropyl alcohol into each ear canal to be treated; wait 45 seconds
   c. Flush out the ear canal(s) twice with nonbacteriostatic saline by rotating the head from side to side (failing to flush out alcohol adequately will result in aspiration of alcohol)
   d. Wick out any excess fluid with a cotton swab; can also use suction catheter

2. Reexamine the ear(s):
   a. Remove remaining debris and cerumen with a curette, sterile cotton swab, Baron metal suction device, or wire loop
   b. Visualize anatomic landmarks
3. Hook up suction/collection system

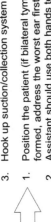

Step 4: Perform tympanocentesis

1. Position the patient (if bilateral tympanocentesis will be performed, address the worst ear first)
2. Assistant should use both hands to firmly stabilize child's head
3. Place gentle traction on the pinna with thumb, insert the otoscope and needle, and point the tip of the needle toward the anterior inferior quadrant, halfway between the tip of the malleus and rim of the ear canal
4. Penetrate tympanic membrane (TM); a slight "pop" may be felt, like sensation felt during lumbar puncture when entering dura
5. As soon as the lumen of the needle enters the TM, stop advancing the needle and cover the hole of the aspirator (in smaller children, the tip of the needle may touch the petrous bone)
6. Keep the trap of the aspirator level as aspirate collects specimen to prevent specimen going into suction machine
7. When all pus has been aspirated (usually 1 to 2 seconds),‡ withdraw the needle
8. Aspirate 0.5 mL of nonbacteriostatic saline through the needle into the trap to clear specimen from needle

Continued

5

79

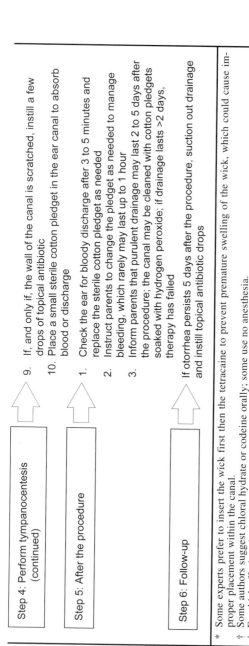

Step 4: Perform tympanocentesis (continued)

9. If, and only if, the wall of the canal is scratched, instill a few drops of topical antibiotic
10. Place a small sterile cotton pledget in the ear canal to absorb blood or discharge

Step 5: After the procedure

1. Check the ear for bloody discharge after 3 to 5 minutes and replace the sterile cotton pledget as needed
2. Instruct parents to change the pledget as needed to manage bleeding, which rarely may last up to 1 hour
3. Inform parents that purulent drainage may last 2 to 5 days after the procedure; the canal may be cleaned with cotton pledgets soaked with hydrogen peroxide; if drainage lasts >2 days, therapy has failed

Step 6: Follow-up

If otorrhea persists 5 days after the procedure, suction out drainage and instill topical antibiotic drops

* Some experts prefer to insert the wick first then the tetracaine to prevent premature swelling of the wick, which could cause improper placement within the canal.
† Some authors suggest chloral hydrate or codeine orally; some use no anesthesia.
‡ For thick effusions it may be necessary to alternate pressure/suction by covering and uncovering the thumb-hole of the aspirator. If the effusion is still too thick to aspirate, make a second puncture a few millimeters posterior to the first. In extreme cases, remove thick fluid by touching the opening in the TM with a large-bore Baron suction instrument under full pressure. If material remains in a strand as you remove the needle, twirl the strand around a sterile cotton swab or Calgiswab and use this to inoculate culture plates.

Adapted from Block SL. *Contemporary Pediatrics.* 1999;16:103-127.

- Streaking plates, placing in a candle jar or CO_2 bag, then incubating.
- Checking plates the next day. If there is no growth, reincubate overnight.
- For plates with growth, inoculate growth onto transport media or chocolate agar slants and submit to a reference laboratory for identification and antibiotic susceptibility testing.
- If lab is available within the office/clinic complex so that <2 hours elapse until sample is in lab, send sealed trap for culture. Otherwise use transport media (see above), but yield will be reduced.

For next-day presumptive identification of pneumococcus and its susceptibility or resistance to penicillin, optochin and oxacillin disks may be dropped onto the initial blood agar plates if clinicians are able to perform basic microbiology.

Efficacy of Tympanocentesis

Tympanocentesis should only be performed when a purulent MEE is assured. Therefore, for the inexperienced clinician, it may be advisable to utilize tympanometry or acoustic reflectometry (see Chapter 4, *Diagnosis*) prior to tympanocentesis to confirm the presence of an MEE. However, both instruments may give a normal reading in 10% to 20% of children with a bona fide purulent MEE.[4] Using the AAP/AAFP guideline as criteria for a purulent MEE will be inadequate, as the guideline allows any type of MEE (AOM, otitis media with effusion [OME], and eustachian tube dysfunction) plus nonspecific symptoms to be considered as AOM. Instead, practitioners will want to use the criteria of AOM set forth in this book before considering tympanocentesis.

The rate for recovery of otopathogens from tympanocentesis aspirate is critically dependent on technique. Meticulous technique and immediate inoculation onto solid culture media (sheep blood agar and chocolate agar) have yielded bacteria recovery rates as high as 87% to 95%. The recovery of pathogens from the ears of children who received antibiotics within a few days of the procedure is reduced to about 50%.[1] Some experts also inoculate broth medium with the same swab used to inoculate agar. Recovery rates are reduced when a commercial transport medium is used and when the culture is incubated for an extended period at room temperature. The bacteria recovery rate will also be reduced if:

- Alcohol is used to sterilize the external canal and solution remaining in the canal is not rinsed out thoroughly
- Residual tetracaine is not thoroughly rinsed out
- If a concentration of tetracaine >8% is used, rate of bacterial recovery is greatly reduced.

Tetracaine's anesthetic effect on the TM persists for 30 to 60 minutes.

Safety of Tympanocentesis

Most experienced otoscopists report no serious complications of tympanocentesis (never observed by either author), but the following complications are possible[1]:

- Chronic TM perforation (much less risk than with insertion of a tympanostomy tube)
- Bleeding from accidentally piercing the internal bulb of the jugular vein (in one case, minor oozing lasted about 30 minutes; usually bleeding stops in minutes with a cotton ball inserted into the canal for tamponade)

- Piercing the oval window (this should not occur if the proper area of the TM is punctured)
- Disruption of the ossicles, with possible hearing loss (this should not occur when the practitioner knows and obtains good visualization of anatomic landmarks and restrains the child firmly)
- Permanent hearing loss (unless ossicles are disrupted, draining the abscess actually improves the temporary hearing loss that accompanies AOM and decreases the risk of permanent hearing loss due to long-standing infection)
- Facial nerve paralysis (tympanocentesis is the recommended therapy for AOM with facial paralysis and poses no more risk of injury to an abnormally located facial nerve than does pressure equalizing [PE] tube placement).

REFERENCES

1. Block SL. Tympanocentesis: why, when, how. *Contemporary Pediatrics*. 1999;16:103-127.

2. American Academy of Pediatrics Subcommittee on Management of Acute Otitis Media. Diagnosis and management of acute otitis media. *Pediatrics*. 2004;113:1451-1465.

3. Dowell SF, Butler JC, Giebink GS, et al. Acute otitis media: management and surveillance in an era of pneumococcal resistance-a report from the Drug-Resistant *Streptococcus pneumoniae* Therapeutic Working Group. *Pediatr Infect Dis J*. 1999;18:1-9.

4. Block SL, Pichichero ME, McLinn S, Aronovitz G, Kimball S. Spectral gradient acoustic reflectometry: detection of middle ear effusion in suppurative acute otitis media. *Pediatr Infect Dis J*. 1999;18:741-744.

6 Basis for Antibiotic Selection

Selecting the optimal antibiotic with which to treat acute otitis media (AOM) became much more difficult during the 1990s. This was due to dramatically increased prevalence of traditional AOM pathogens with higher rates of resistance to traditional antibiotics. For example, in the past (1990s)[1]:

- *Penicillin-nonsusceptible Streptococcus pneumoniae* (PNSP) was recovered in up to 50% of nonrefractory AOM.
- PNSP strains were being recovered in 50% to 90% of *S pneumoniae* isolates in cases of refractory AOM from some geographic locations.
- Resistance of *S pneumoniae* to oral cephalosporins paralleled or exceeded resistance to penicillin.
- In the United States, β-lactamase–producing strains of *Haemophilus influenzae* and *Moraxella catarrhalis* were being recovered in nearly 50% and 100%, respectively, of strains from AOM.
- 50% to 70% of *H influenzae* was resistant to newer macrolides.
- Up to 30% of penicillin-susceptible *S pneumoniae* (PSSP) was resistant to trimethoprim-sulfamethoxazole (TMP/SMX).
- >90% of PNSP was resistant to TMP/SMX.

The 2000s: Pneumococcal Conjugate Vaccine Era AOM Studies

In the decade of the 2000s, a marked shift in the microbiology of AOM in the United States has occurred due to routine use of pneumococcal conjugate vaccine (PCV)–7. In the United States where PCV-7 has been available since March 2000, a shift in the microbiology of AOM has occurred over the years within populations and/or children who have received adequate doses of PCV-7 during early childhood or infancy. These studies from distinctly different demographic populations have shown a marked proportional shift toward gram-negative pathogens and a reduction in *S pneumoniae* in young children who have received PCV-7.

Four studies have documented some of these changes in AOM:

- Eskola study (Finland)[2]
- Block study (rural Kentucky)[3]
- Casey and Pichichero study (Rochester, NY)[4]
- Caspary study (Norfolk, Virginia).[5]

■ Eskola Study (Finland)

In the first clinical trials in Finland examining the microbiology of AOM after PCV-7 (1995-1997) where the population at large was not vaccinated, 1662 children ages 6 to 24 months who developed AOM underwent tympanocentesis.[2] The authors observed an overall 6% reduction of AOM and a 34% reduction in overall pneumococcal episodes of AOM. AOM specifically due to vaccine serotypes of *S pneumoniae* decreased by 57%. They also noted a 31% increase in rates of *H influenzae* among PCV-7 vaccinees, and AOM due to non–PCV-7 types also increased (the latter is termed "serotype substitution").

NOTE: Each of the following studies examined primarily or exclusively children who had either refractory or recurrent AOM and who were mostly <24 months of age. Thus we do not have any significant data on the microbiology of new-onset AOM for PCV-7 children.

■ Block Study (Rural Kentucky)

These investigators studied the microbiology of AOM among children 7 to 24 months of age who had each received PCV-7 in a rural Kentucky population. The patient population consisted of[3]:

- 100% of study subjects were <24 months and all were vaccinated with three or four doses of PCV-7 (94% of all young children attending this clinic were also vaccinated with PCV-7, providing the possibility for a herd-immunity effect)
- 76% of the post–PCV-7 population had received antibiotics within the last 30 days (vs 59% in the pre–PCV-7 group; *P* value)
- 78% of the post–PCV-7 population was otitis prone (vs 43% in the pre–PCV-7 group; *P* value)
- 65% of the post–PCV-7 group attended day care (vs 29% in the pre–PCV-7 population; *P* value).

This comparative study showed a major shift in the microbiology of AOM: *S pneumoniae* decreased from 48% to 31% (a 36% reduction) and nontypeable *H influenzae* increased from 41% to 56% (a 34% increase) (**Figure 6.1**). Gram-negative and β-lactamase pathogens accounted for nearly two thirds and one half, respectively, of all AOM pathogens recovered in children receiving three or four doses of PCV-7. PNSP and high-level resistant PNSP accounted for 19% and 5%, respectively, of all AOM pathogens recovered among PCV-7 children.

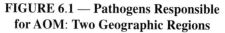

FIGURE 6.1 — Pathogens Responsible for AOM: Two Geographic Regions

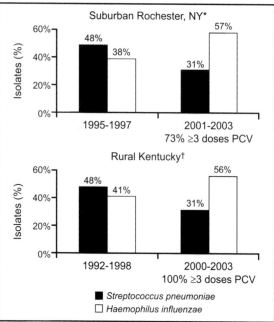

Abbreviations: AOM, acute otitis media; PCV, pneumococcal conjugate vaccine.

Recurrent AOM or AOM treatment failure. It should be noted that Rochester had 100% recurrent or persistent AOM.

* Rate of patients ≤24 months of age was 80%.
† Rate of patients ≤24 months of age was 100%.

Casey JR, Pichichero ME. *Pediatr Infect Dis J.* 2004;23:824-828; Block SL, et al. *Pediatr Infect Dis J.* 2004;23:829-833.

The proportion of vaccine-related serotypes 6A and 19A also increased from 8% to 32% of *S pneumoniae* strains recovered. Other nonvaccine serotypes did not significantly replace vaccine serotypes or PNSP strains in this population.

■ Casey and Pichichero Study (Rochester, NY)

Among children in a 1998-2000 cohort, when high-dose amoxicillin had become the standard therapy, the marked proportional shift toward *H influenzae* was not noted.[4] Only after PCV-7 was routinely used in this population did the proportion of *H influenzae* increase from 38% (1995-1997) to 57% (2001-2003) of all AOM pathogens recovered—nearly identical to the phenomenon observed in the rural Kentucky population (**Figure 6.1**). This was an impressive study with a convincingly large number of patients (551 children). Seventy-two percent of the children in the study were <24 months of age; 73% has three or four doses of PCV-7 in the 2001-2003 group. All children in the study had persistent or recurrent AOM. There was a 24% decrease in office visits from pre–PCV-7 in the PCV-7 group. The difference in rates from 1995-1996 to 2001-2003, respectively, for all AOM pathogens were:

- *H influenzae*:
  - β-lactamase negative: 38% vs 57% (+50%)
  - β-lactamase positive: 46% vs 55%
- *S pneumoniae*: 48% vs 31% (−35%)
- PNSP: 24% vs 10%.

■ Caspary Study (Norfolk, Virginia)
(Chronic otitis media study [undergoing tympanostomy tube insertion])

Caspary and colleagues compared the bacteriology recovered from two cohorts of children from 2001-2002 undergoing tympanostomy tube insertion.[5] In looking only at the PCV-7 vs non–PCV-7 cohorts in 2001-2002, the median ages of the children were 14 months in the PCV-7 group and 24 months in the non–PCV-7 group. A total of 127 (28%) of 446 patients grew at least one organism of which:

- 52% were *H influenzae* (69% and 43%, respectively)
- 28% were *M catarrhalis* (22% and 32%, respectively)
- 12% were *S pneumoniae* (11% and 12%, respectively).

The rates of *H influenzae* and *S pneumoniae* were 65% and 38%, respectively, in a cohort from the same practice in 1996-1997 as reported by Sutton and colleagues.[6] Comparing PCV-7–vaccinated to unvaccinated children, *H influenzae* was nearly 3-fold more likely to be recovered. These data show that PNSP has become uncommon in low-acuity AOM or in otitis media with effusion (OME) and that *S pneumoniae* accounts for only ~10% of organisms isolated among children undergoing tympanostomy tube placement.

NOTE: In each of these studies of young children, most of whom had received PCV-7, *H influenzae* had become the predominant pathogen of AOM. Less than 20% of pathogens recovered in the studies from US investigators were PNSP. Only 5% to 6% of all middle ear pathogens were highly resistant PNSP among children with refractory/recurrent AOM.

Vaccine Serotype Replacement After PCV-7

Block and colleagues' data showed that serotypes 6A and 19A proportionately account for almost one third of pneumococcal strains recovered in AOM vs 8% pre–PCV-7.[3] They also found that PCV-7 serotypes accounted for 70% and 36% of isolates pre–PCV-7 vs post–PCV-7, respectively. In this population, herd immunity was likely occurring due to the very high rates of PCV-7 vaccination. Because of the absolute decrease in the rates of vaccine serotypes, these data suggest that the increased rate of nonvaccine serotypes is more likely a proportional increase, not an absolute increase.

McEllistrem and associates studied a population of children in the Pittsburgh area.[7] They found a proportion of nonvaccine serogroups causing AOM increased from 14.8% (13 of 88) in 1999 to 36.5% (22 of 63) in 2001. They did not specifically serotype their organisms.

Eskola and colleagues enrolled 1662 infants in a randomized, double-blind efficacy trial of a heptavalent pneumococcal polysaccharide conjugate vaccine. The number of episodes attributed to serotypes that are cross-reactive with those in the vaccine was reduced by 51%, whereas the number of episodes due to all other serotypes increased by 33%.[2]

Choices for Antibiotic Therapy for AOM

Current choices for antibiotic therapy for AOM in young children include 16 oral-suspension formulations and one intramuscular antibiotic (**Table 6.1**). First, clinicians need to consider the bacteriology of AOM — which type of pathogen is likely to be present (for example, *S pneumoniae* or nontypeable *H influenzae*) and what is the likelihood of resistance to antibiotics. If several drugs appear comparable in bacterial coverage, the clinician should consider the following:

- Managed-care formulary
- Concomitant coinfection
- Gastrointestinal (GI) distress
- Palatability
- Dosing frequency.

TABLE 6.1 — Antibiotics Available for the Treatment of Acute Otitis Media in Young Children

Antibiotic Class/Agent	Trade Name	Total Daily Dose*	Dosing Schedule(s)
Penicillins			
Amoxicillin	Amoxil, Wymox,	<3 and >36 mo: 40-60 mg/kg	>36 mo: 20-30 mg/kg q 12h × 10 d
		3-36 mo or suspect PNSP: 80-90 mg/kg	3-36 mo: 40-45 mg/kg q 12h × 10 d; maximum daily dose is 3 g
Amoxicillin/clavulanate	Augmentin	45/6.4 mg/kg (≥2 mo)	22.5/3.2 mg q12h × 10 d
	Augmentin ES-600	90/6.4 mg/kg	45/3.2 mg q12h × 10 d
Cephalosporins			
Second-Generation			
Cefaclor	Ceclor	30 mg/kg (6 mo-12 y)	15 mg/kg q12h × 10 d
Cefprozil	Cefzil	30 mg/kg (6 mo-12 y)	15 mg/kg q12h × 10 d
Cefuroxime axetil	Ceftin	30 mg/kg (3 mo-12 y/33 kg)	15 mg/kg q12h × 10 d
Loracarbef	Lorabid	30 mg/kg (6 mo-12 y)	15 mg/kg q12h × 10 d

Third-Generation			
Cefdinir	Omnicef	14 mg/kg (6 mo-12 y/43 kg)	14 mg/kg q24h × 10 d[†]
Cefixime	Suprax	8 mg/kg (6 mo-12 y/50 kg)	8 mg/kg q24h × 10 d
Cefpodoxime proxetil	Vantin	10 mg/kg (2 mo-12 y/40 kg)	10 mg/kg/d × 10 d[†]
Ceftibuten	Cedax	9 mg/kg (6 mo-12 y/45 kg)	9 mg/kg q24h × 10 d
Ceftriaxone	Rocephin	50 mg/kg	Single dose[‡]
Macrolides			
Azithromycin	Zithromax	10, 5, 5, 5 mg/kg (≥6 mo)	q24h × 5 d
		10, 10, 10 mg/kg	q24h × 3 d
		30 mg/kg	Single dose
Clarithromycin	Biaxin	15 mg/kg (≥6 mo)	7.5 mg/kg q12h × 10 d
Other			
Clindamycin[†]	Cleocin	30 mg/kg	10 mg/kg tid

Continued

6

Antibiotic Class/Agent	Trade Name	Total Daily Dose*	Dosing Schedule(s)
Combinations			
Erythromycin/sulfisoxazole	Pediazole	50/160 mg/kg	Divided qid or tid
Trimethoprim/sulfamethoxazole	Septra/Bactrim	8/40 mg/kg (≥2 mo)	4/20 mg/kg q12h × 10 d

Abbreviation: PNSP, penicillin non-susceptible *Streptococcus pneumoniae*.

* Patient weight or age guidelines are used for determining dosage.
† Also approved by the Food and Drug Administration (FDA) for 5 days when treating uncomplicated acute otitis media (AOM). Authors prefer this treatment protocol only in those patients >2 years of age.
‡ For refractory AOM, single dose q 24 hr × 3 days. See text for alternative approach.

Physicians' Desk Reference. 59th ed. Montvale, NJ: Medical Economics Company; 2005.

If several drugs remain viable options, the narrowest-spectrum drug is preferred.

Bacteriology of AOM

The pathogens and their drug susceptibilities in a given case of AOM can only be determined by obtaining a specimen of middle ear effusion (MEE) by tympanocentesis and performing a culture or culturing recent-onset (<48 hours) otorrhea. The following factors may influence the bacteriology of AOM:

- Use of PCV-7 vaccine
  - Individual (number and proximity of doses)
  - Community (>88% may give herd immunity)
- Type of AOM (new onset vs refractory)
- Season
- Geographic location
- Patient age
- Day care attendance
- Sibling with PNSP[8]
- Recent antibiotics.

A limited alternative to middle ear culture is nasopharyngeal culture, which is only a negative predictor in AOM. The lack of antibiotic-resistant pathogens in deep nasopharyngeal cultures (>95%) predicts that the AOM pathogen will not be antibiotic resistant as well.[9] Nasopharyngeal surveillance cultures may also provide a surrogate marker in AOM as to the prevalence of *S pneumoniae* serotypes. As an example, Pelton and colleagues studied two Boston communities in 2000-2003 and found that PCV-7 produced a marked decline in vaccine serotypes carried in the nasopharynx of young children (from 22% to 2%).[10] Commensurately, nonvaccine serotypes increased from 7% to 16%.

■ Mechanisms of Antibiotic Resistance

Table 6.1 shows antibiotic classes currently available to treat AOM. The classes reflect different mechanisms of antibiotic action:

- Gram-negative strains of nontypeable *H influenzae* and *M catarrhalis* develop resistance to penicillins, cephalosporins, and other β-lactam drugs by producing β-lactamases, enzymes that hydrolyze the β-lactam structure that is key to drug action.

- Drug-resistant strains of *S pneumoniae* have acquired genes that produce altered penicillin-binding proteins (PBPs) in the cell wall producing resistance to penicillins and cephalosporins.[11] Other major genes have been identified for macrolide resistance:

  - The erythromycin ribosomal methylation (erm) gene codes (associated with resistant PNSP [PNSP-R] correlates with high-level resistance (minimum inhibitory concentration [MIC] >16 mg/L) to azithromycin, clindamycin, and ketolides (eg, telithromycin, which is approved for adult respiratory infections).

  - The macrolide efflux pump (mef) associated with the intermediate PNSP gene produces proteins that serve as antibiotic efflux pumps for macrolides. Presence of the mef gene usually confers a low level of resistance (MIC 2-8 mg/L) that theoretically may be overcome by higher concentration of drug (associated with intermediate PNSP [PNSP-I]). Mutants of mef are susceptible to clindamycin and telithromycin

- Alteration of folic acid pathway enzymes conveys resistance to trimethoprim and sulfonamide drugs.

- Efflux pumps have recently been described in *H influenzae* for macrolides and azithromycin
- Quinolone resistance (<5% of pneumococci and *H influenzae*) is conveyed by mutations in DNA gyrase or topoisomerase (enzymes needed to package newly made DNA into the next generation of replicating bacteria).

■ Measuring Antibiotic Susceptibilities of AOM Pathogens

Pathogen susceptibility to an antibiotic can be measured and expressed in various ways:

- Dilution techniques (broth, agar, microdilution, etc) measure the MIC of drug (mg/L) needed to achieve inhibition of growth of the pathogen in culture (**Figure 6.2**).
- Diffusion techniques (such as E test) involve culturing the AOM pathogen(s) with antibiotic impregnated strips that contain measured amounts of each antibiotic to be tested. Susceptibility can also be determined by disk-diffusion methods (Kirby-Bauer) as the diameter (in millimeters) of the zone of inhibition of pathogen growth.

Subcultures of the MEE isolates are tested with concentrations of the antibiotic(s) of interest. To help clinicians interpret the results of drug-susceptibility testing, the Clinical and Laboratory Standards Institute (CLSI) National Committee on Clinical Laboratory Standards (NCCLS) periodically tests and reports the susceptibility break points (for both dilution and diffusion techniques) of aerobic bacteria for various antibiotics. As an example, when broth microdilution is used to assay the penicillin resistance of an isolate of *S pneumoniae* from MEE, the isolate is considered:

- Resistant (highly resistant) to penicillin if its MIC is >2.0 mg/L

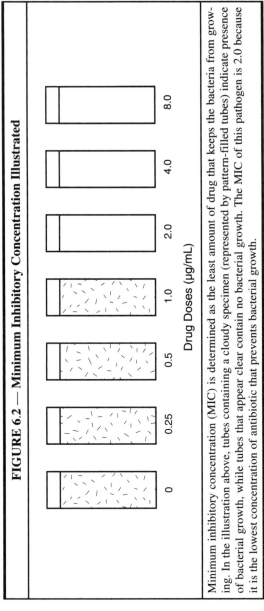

FIGURE 6.2 — Minimum Inhibitory Concentration Illustrated

Drug Doses (μg/mL)

0   0.25   0.5   1.0   2.0   4.0   8.0

Minimum inhibitory concentration (MIC) is determined as the least amount of drug that keeps the bacteria from growing. In the illustration above, tubes containing a cloudy specimen (represented by pattern-filled tubes) indicate presence of bacterial growth, while tubes that appear clear contain no bacterial growth. The MIC of this pathogen is 2.0 because it is the lowest concentration of antibiotic that prevents bacterial growth.

- Intermediately resistant if its MIC is 0.1 to <2 mg/L
- Susceptible to penicillin if its MIC is <0.1 mg/L.

Table 6.2 summarizes the most recent CLSI susceptibility break points established by broth microdilution of *S pneumoniae* and *H influenzae* for antibiotics currently used to treat AOM.[12]

■ Overall Prevalence of AOM Bacterial Pathogens

The prevalence of AOM caused by various pathogens has been identified by culturing samples of MEE obtained by tympanocentesis. Because of differences in the demographics of populations studied and the techniques used to obtain and culture specimens, the rate and type of bacteria recovered vary somewhat. Overall, however, bacteria have been recovered from 65% to 95% of aspirates of MEE, depending on the technique.[1]

The four major types of bacteria that have been isolated in AOM from studies worldwide are *S pneumoniae*, nontypeable *H influenzae*, *M catarrhalis* (or Branhamella), and group A Streptococcus.[13-15]

Two or three pathogens may be cultured simultaneously from a small proportion (usually <10%) of MEE isolates.[13,16,17] *Streptococcus pyogenes* is a more common pathogen in older children, accounting for 8% to 16% of isolates.[18]

Atypical pathogens in AOM have been reported, including the following:
- *Chlamydia pneumoniae*, a common cause of pediatric pneumonia, was first cultured in MEE from otherwise healthy children with AOM in 1997. The pathogen was present in 8% of MEE from 101 children with AOM, but it was the sole pathogen in only two cases. All eight children

TABLE 6.2 — Current NCCLS Susceptibility Break Points* of *Streptococcus pneumoniae* and *Haemophilus influenzae* for Oral Suspension and Injectable Antibiotic Therapeutic Agents for Acute Otitis Media[†]

Antibiotic Agent	S pneumoniae	H influenzae
Penicillins[†]		
Amoxicillin	≤2	≤1
Amoxicillin/clavulanate	≤2/1[‡]	≤4/2[‡]
Cephalosporins[†]		
Second-Generation		
Cefaclor/Loracarbef	≤2	≤8
Cefprozil	≤2	≤8
Cefuroxime axetil	≤1	≤4
Third-Generation[†]		
Cefdinir	≤0.5	≤1

Cefixime	≤2	≤1
Cefpodoxime	≤0.5	≤2
Ceftibuten (parenteral)§	≤0.06	≤2
Ceftriaxone	≤1.0, ≥4.0‖	≤2
Macrolides†		
Azithromycin	≤0.5	≤4
Clarithromycin	≤0.25	≤8
Quinolones		
Ciprofloxacin	NA	≤1
Gatifloxacin	≤1	≤1
Levofloxacin	≤2	≤2
Ofloxacin	≤2	≤2
Other		
Clindamycin§	≤0.25	NA

Continued

Antibiotic Agent	S pneumoniae	H influenzae
Combinations		
Erythromycin/sulfisoxazole[§]	NA	≤0.5
Trimethoprim/sulfamethoxazole[§]	≤0.5	≤0.5

Abbreviations: NA, not available for individual organisms, susceptibility given is for most organisms; NCCLS, National Committee on Clinical Laboratory Standards.

* Broth dilution (MIC in µg/mL).

† Data from the NCCLS. Methods for Dilution Antimicrobial Susceptibility Tests for Bacteria That Grow Aerobically; Approved Standard – ed 5. M7-A5; vol 22, no 1, Jan 2002.

‡ Augmentin ES-600/Augmentin standard dose (45 mg/kg/d).

§ Data from the NCCLS publication Methods for Dilution Antimicrobial Susceptibility Tests for Bacteria That Grow Aerobically (3rd ed). Villanova, Pa: NCCLS, 1993, reported in *Physicians' Desk Reference.* 59th ed. Montvale, NJ: Medical Economics Company; 2005.

‖ These values apply to middle ear effusion and other nonmeningitis isolates: ≤1.0 = susceptible; 2.0 = intermediate; ≥4.0 = resistant. For meningitis, <1.0 = susceptible; 1.0 = intermediate; ≥2.0 = resistant.

with *C pneumoniae* were younger than 60 months and five were younger than 16 months of age.[19]

- *Chlamydia trachomatis* has rarely been cultured in AOM.[19] Indirect detection with fluorescent antibody staining does not differentiate it from *C pneumoniae*.
- *Mycoplasma pneumoniae* rarely causes AOM or even bullous myringitis (**Color Plate 1**, **F**).

■ Bacteriology of Persistent/Recurrent AOM

The bacteriology of AOM differs depending on the type of AOM present, as demonstrated by the results of studies by Harrison and colleagues,[20] Del Beccaro and colleagues,[21] and a review by Pichichero.[22] Pichichero examined children with recurrent AOM in 1995-1996 and observed that of 89 *S pneumoniae* isolates, 13% were PNSP-I and 35% were PNSP-R. Of 71 *H influenzae* strains, 58% were β-lactamase–positive.[23]

1980s Pathogens

Before PNSP in AOM was known to be widespread in the United States, Harrison and colleagues recovered *S pneumoniae* or group A streptococcus less frequently from recently treated AOM. They recovered multiple organisms (*Staphylococcus aureus* and *H influenzae* [including β-lactamase–producing organisms]) more frequently from the MEE of recently treated AOM. PNSP-I made up 18% of these *S pneumoniae* cases from the early 1980s. They also found that approximately 50% of isolates taken from recently treated ears were susceptible to the antibiotic prescribed for the previous episode, suggesting that factors other than antimicrobial susceptibility are important in the occurrence of persistent/refractory/recurrent AOM.[20]

1990s Pathogens

During the 1990s, Block and colleagues found that PNSP was 5-fold more frequent in children who had recently received antibiotics (within 3 days) than in those who had not received antibiotics within 3 days.[16] Among all pathogens recovered from the antibiotic-failure group, they found PNSP-R, 30%; PNSP-I, 14%; and penicillin-susceptible *S pneumoniae* (PSSP), 37%. In contrast, among those not treated within 3 days, they found PNSP-R, 2%; PNSP-I, 7%; and PSSP, 39%.

2000s Pathogens: PCV-7 Data

During the 2000s among children who have received PCV-7, *H influenzae* now accounts for more than half of the organisms of AOM, and in fact appears to be 2-fold more common than *S pneumoniae* among young children who have refractory/recurrent AOM.[3,4] Gram-negative organisms account for almost two thirds of pathogens in the middle ear. Between 55% and 64% of *H influenzae* isolates in AOM were β-lactamase producers. PNSP now accounts for <20% of all AOM pathogens in refractory/recurrent AOM.

■ Time Period and Likelihood of Antibiotic Resistance

Amoxicillin, in traditional doses (40 mg/kg/day divided tid), had been reasonably effective in treating AOM due to the most frequent AOM pathogens (*S pneumoniae*, *H influenzae*, and *M catarrhalis*) until the 1990s, when AOM caused by PNSP became widespread in the United States.[14] β-Lactamase–producing nontypeable *H influenzae* resistant to amoxicillin became relatively common in the mid to late 1970s. β-lactamase–producing strains of *M catarrhalis* were also identified in recent decades, and has been nearly 100% β-lactamase producing for over 2 decades. From the 1980s to the 1990s, there have been an overall increase in the prevalence of AOM caused by strains of AOM pathogens resistant to multiple antibiotics (referred to as drug-resistant strains), eg, PNSP-R, as shown in **Table 6.3**.[1]

Even more notable increases in resistance have recently developed to other classes of drugs. For example, resistance to TMP/SMX has risen from 13% to 30% in PSSP respiratory isolates in children and >95% resistance in PNSP isolates. Resistance rates to TMP/SMX for *H influenzae* have reached approximately 25% to 30% as well. Since 1999, resistance to macrolides/azalides has risen to about 45% of PNSP and 45% to 70% for all strains of *H influenzae* in one area. However, the routine macrolide use in a community may also be related to some slight decreases in resistance to macrolides, as fewer strains of PNSP account for the total number of *S pneumoniae* isolates. For example, in the Boston area since PCV-7, rates of antibiotic resistance of *S pneumoniae* isolates to penicillin and azithromycin were 29.3% and 26.5%, respectively.[10] First- and second-generation quinolones have shown no resistance among *H influenzae* isolates, but approximately 50% resistance was noted among PNSP isolates during the mid-1990s, particularly among drugs such as ciprofloxacin and ofloxacin. While resistance to levofloxacin has been increasing as well, it remains <5% in general. Resistance to gatifloxacin and moxifloxacin remains <1% in most areas. Thus all classes of drugs currently appear to have resistance problems, some more than others. For more details on antibiotic resistance, see Chapter 8, *Second-Line and Third-Line Antibiotic Therapy*.

The prevalence of drug-resistant AOM has also been shown to vary from one time to the next in the same population.[17]

TABLE 6.3 — Proportions of Resistant Pathogens Causing Nonrefractory Acute Otitis Media in US Children During the 1980s, 1990s, and 2000s

Pathogen	Approximate Proportion of All Pathogens Recovered (%)		
	1980s	**1990s**	**2000s**
Haemophilus influenzae (nontypeable)			
β-Lactamase(−)	30	10	15
β-Lactamase(+)	10	20	35
Moraxella catarrhalis			
β-Lactamase(−)	5	0	0
β-Lactamase(+)	5	10	0
Total of all β-lactamase(+)	15	30	45
Streptococcus pneumoniae			
Penicillin susceptible	48	35	20
Penicillin nonsusceptible	2	15	10

For more details on antibiotic resistance to other classes of antimicrobials, many of which have equal or more resistance than penicillins, see Chapter 8, *Second-Line and Third-Line Antibiotic Therapy.* Increased doses of penicillins (amoxicillin or penicillin) may produce clinical success in treating "resistant" pneumococcal infections outside the central nervous system because resistance that is based on altered penicillin-binding proteins is not absolute but only relative to the amount of penicillin at the infection site. However, this same higher-dose strategy does not increase success for amoxicillin when treating β-lactamase–producing *H influenzae.*

Block SL, Pichichero ME. *Pediatr Infect Dis J.* 2004;23:829-833; Casey JR, et al. *Pediatr Infect Dis J.* 2004;23:824-828.

6

■ Geographic Location and Likelihood of Antibiotic Resistance

Geographic location affects the prevalence of AOM due to antibiotic-resistant pathogens. As a result, clinicians need to consider current trends in antibiotic susceptibility among respiratory isolates in children from their area. For example, a 1997 surveillance study of the susceptibilities of isolates from six regions of the United States to 10 antimicrobial drugs is shown in **Figure 6.3**.[24] Nationwide, the surveillance study found resistance among 50% of *S pneumoniae* isolates and 42% of *H influenzae* isolates from the middle ears and nasopharynges of children and the sinuses of adults. The prevalence of antibiotic-resistant isolates of these pathogens varied somewhat by region.[24]

■ Patient Age and Likelihood of Antibiotic Resistance

Several studies found that younger patients, particularly those younger than 24 months, are more likely to have more episodes of AOM and more episodes that are persistent or recurrent. They also tend to have a higher frequency of drug-resistant pathogens.[14,16,24-26]

With the use of PCV-7 in the routine immunization schedule, the susceptibility of *S pneumoniae* isolates in North America from 2001-2002 from children ages 0 to 5 has improved. For example, for *S pneumoniae*, the rate of resistance to two oral cephalosporin antibiotics and penicillin have been reduced by 6% and 8%, respectively. Overall, there has been a slight reduction in the proportion of PNSP from 2001 to 2002 among all age groups (**Table 6.4**).[27]

■ Day Care and Likelihood of Antibiotic Resistance

Day care attendance is a major risk factor for recurrent AOM and antibiotic-resistant AOM:

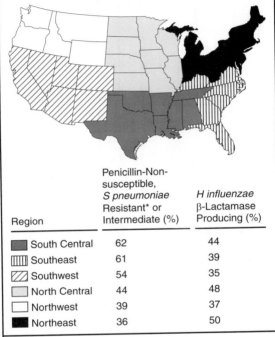

FIGURE 6.3 — Regional Variation in Percentage of Resistant Strains of *Streptococcus pneumoniae* and *Haemophilus influenzae**†

Region	Penicillin-Non-susceptible, *S pneumoniae* Resistant* or Intermediate (%)	*H influenzae* β-Lactamase Producing (%)
South Central	62	44
Southeast	61	39
Southwest	54	35
North Central	44	48
Northwest	39	37
Northeast	36	50

* Includes adults and children.
† Percentages are prior to the routine use of pneumococcal conjugate vaccine-7.

Jacobs MR, et al. *Antimicrob Agents Chemother.* 1999;43:1901-1908.

- Nasopharyngeal carriage rates as high as 53% for PNSP-R and 22% for PNSP-I have been reported in children enrolled in day care in the United States.[28]
- When otitis-prone condition and number of antibiotic courses were excluded, another study

TABLE 6.4 — Change in the Rate of Penicillin Resistance Among *Streptococcus pneumoniae* Isolates From North America (2001 to 2002) Listed by Patient Age Group*

Age Group (Years)	Intermediate (%)			Resistant (%)		
	2001	2002	Variation	2001	2002	Variation
0–5	16.8	16.8	0.0	34.4	28.1	–6.3
6–64	15.2	14.7	–0.5	18.5	13.8	–4.7
≥65	11.7	10.4	–1.3	23.0	16.0	–7.0

* All strains were from respiratory tract infections.

Sader HS, et al. *Diagn Microbiol Infect Dis.* 2003;47:515-525.

showed that day care attendance increases the risk for AOM caused by PNSP by 2.3-fold.[16]

- Having a sibling with PNSP is also a risk for PNSP[8,28]
- The rate of AOM due to PNSP in children younger than 6 years who were not otitis prone was 42% for those in day care compared with only 24% for those not in day care.[29]

PNSP in AOM still presents a significant clinical challenge in the early 21st century because:

- *S pneumoniae* remains the most prevalent AOM pathogen worldwide; however, in the United States with the use of PCV-7, the rates of *S pneumoniae* organisms in AOM and in invasive disease have declined by about 50% and 69%, respectively, in children <2 years of age.[3,4,30] The original Kaiser-Permanente study showed 87% and 58% reduction in invasive disease caused by vaccine serotypes in the <1-year-old and <2-year-old age groups, respectively. It appears that AOM due to PNSP has also markedly decreased as a result of herd immunity now that there have been several years of uniform routine PCV-7 use in communities.[3,4]
- Localized *S pneumoniae* infection can sometimes lead to invasive disease, but local nontypeable *H influenzae* and *M catarrhalis* infections rarely invade.[28]
- The proportion of β-lactamase–positive *H influenzae* or *M catarrhalis* accounts for over half of all AOM organisms among PCV-7 children in 2000.[3-5,25]
- Resistance of *S pneumoniae* to β-lactam drugs persists. But since the introduction of PCV-7 in the vaccine schedule for US children, rates of resistance to β-lactam antibiotics in microbiologic surveys have shown a slight reversal.[11]

111

Nonetheless, a >90% reduction in invasive disease (sepsis, meningitis) from *S pneumoniae* can be attributed to universal use of PCV-7 in the United States. Additionally, the nasopharyngeal carriage of PNSP has similarly decreased to a lesser extent (~50%). Of some concern has been a recent upsurge in 19a, 33, and 11 serotype serous and middle ear disease in isolates from the laboratory of one of the authors. Only time will tell whether this is a temporary phenomenon or the beginning of a new trend.

Adverse Effects and Patient Compliance With Antibiotic Therapy

When more than one antibiotic appears to provide coverage for likely pathogen(s) in an episode of AOM, the clinician should next consider drug and patient compliance factors. Factors affecting patient/caregiver compliance include adverse effects such as:

- Adverse gastrointestinal (GI) effects
- Cost/managed care coverage
- Palatability
- Dosing schedule
- Duration of therapy.

The potential benefits of a more potent antibiotic may sometimes be outweighed by such factors.

■ Safety and Side Effects

All antibiotics used in the treatment of AOM have been associated with diarrhea and other GI side effects. All carry the risk of selection for *Clostridium difficile* and/or pseudomembranous colitis, a risk that may be somewhat higher with clindamycin after several previous courses of antibiotics. Some medications may more frequently cause serious adverse effects[1]:

- Cefaclor has low antimicrobial potency plus the potential to cause serum sickness–like reaction in up to 3.4% of children.
- Although very rare, Stevens-Johnson syndrome has been reported most frequently with TMP/SMX.
- Rates of adverse GI events from amoxicillin/clavulanate are 2-fold higher than those seen with cephalosporins.

In addition to the risk of very rare adverse effects such as anaphylaxis, prescribers should consider what impact an antibiotic's most common side effects and other factors such as cost, palatability, and dosing schedule might have on patient compliance with therapy (**Table 6.5**).

Cost

Cost is often a consideration when choosing an antibiotic. High cost can lead to exclusion of a drug from the formulary of a managed care health insurance plan. Higher cost as a second- or third-tier antibiotic in a formulary can lead to rejection of the prescription at the pharmacy by the parent. It can also lead to patient or caregiver noncompliance with therapy due to:

- Failing to have the prescription filled and not notifying the clinician
- Possibly stopping medication early, when symptoms abate, to save medication for a possible recurrence or for sibling use.

Although we have only personal experience to support this, we prefer to prescribe a suspension formulation for older children up to 12 years of age. Frequently, patients save medication in a pill or tablet formulation. In contrast, when dispensed as a suspension, it carries a warning to discard the unused portion after 10 to 14 days.

TABLE 6.5 — Patient Compliance Factors for Antibiotics Currently Used to Treat Acute Otitis Media in Young Children*

Antibiotic Class/Agent (Daily Dosage)	Side Effects		Cost	Palatability	Divided Dosing Schedule(s)
	Diarrhea	Vomiting/Gastritis			
Penicillins					
Amoxicillin					
Brand (40-60 mg)	+	—	Moderate	Good	bid × 10 d
Generic (pink)	+	—	Low	Fair	bid × 10 d
Generic (yellow)	+	+	Low	Poor	bid × 10 d
High dose† (80-100 mg)	+	—	Moderate	Good	bid × 10 d
Amoxicillin/clavulanate					
Standard dose	++	+	High	Acceptable-fair	bid × 10 d
High dose (90/6.4 mg)	++	+	High‡	Acceptable-fair	bid × 10 d
Cephalosporins					
Second-Generation					
Cefaclor (30 mg)§	+	—	High-very high	Excellent	bid × 10 d

Cefprozil (30 mg)	+	—	High	Good	bid × 10 d
Cefuroxime axetil (30 mg)	+	++	Very high	Poor	bid × 10 d
Loracarbef (30 mg)	+	—	High	Excellent	bid × 10 d
Third-Generation					
Cefdinir (14 mg)	+	—	High‖	Excellent	qd or bid × 5 d
Cefdinir (14 mg)	+	—	High‖	Excellent	qd or bid × 10 d
Cefixime (8 mg)	+	—	High	Excellent	qd or bid × 10 d
Cefpodoxime proxetil (10 mg)	+	++	High‖	Poor	bid × 5 or 10 d
Ceftibuten (9 mg)	+	—	High	Good	qd × 10 d
Ceftriaxone (50 mg)	++	—	High	NA	Single dose
Ceftriaxone (50 mg)	+++	—	Very high	NA	qd × 3 d‖

Continued

Antibiotic Class/Agent (Daily Dosage)	Side Effects		Cost	Palatability	Divided Dosing Schedule(s)
	Diarrhea	Vomiting/Gastritis			
Macrolides					
Azithromycin (10, 5, 5, 5, 5 mg) <15 kg and >15 kg	+	—	Moderate-high	Good	qd × 5 d
Azithromycin (10, 10, 10 mg)	+	—	Moderate-high	Good	qd × 3 d
Azithromycin (30 mg/single dose)	+	+/++	Moderate-high	Good	Single dose
Clarithromycin (15 mg)	+	++	Moderate-high	Fair-poor	bid × 10 d
Others					
Clindamycin[†] (30 mg)	++	++	High	Poor	tid
Erythromycin/sulfisoxazole (50/160 mg)	+	+++	Moderate	Fair	tid × 10 d
Trimethoprim/sulfamethoxazole					
Brand (8/40 mg)	—	—	Moderate	Good	bid × 10 d
Generic (8/40 mg)	—	+	Low	Poor	bid × 10 d

Key: —, 0% to 4%; +, 5% to 10%; ++, 11% to 15%; +++, 16% to 20%

Abbreviations: GI, gastrointestinal; NA, not available.

* Compliance is one part of the decision process and must be balanced against relative drug potency and expected efficacy (see Table 8.4).

† Drug or dosage not included in Food and Drug Administration (FDA) indications for treatment of uncomplicated AOM in children. Caution, as has more than average risk of *Clostridum difficile* diarrhea.

‡ Cost is identical to wholesaler for standard and extra strength (ES) formulations used for standard and high doses, respectively.

§ Cefaclor has been associated with a 3.4% rate of serum sickness–like reaction.

‖ Less expensive if given bid for 5 days, which applies only to children weighing >15 kg (endorsed by AAP/AAFP Guideline).

¶ Three doses are not approved for acute otitis media (AOM) by the FDA, but recommended by the Center for Disease Control (CDC) group. Can be given qd × 3 or qod, the number of total doses depending on persistance of signs/ symptoms. Maximum number of doses not to exceed three.

Physicians' Desk Reference. 59th ed. Montvale, NJ: Medical Economics Company; 2005.

6

Palatability

Children in particular are unlikely to complete a full course of a liquid medication if they find it unpalatable. For ease of administration, suspensions are available for most antibiotics used to treat AOM in children. However, adults participating in a double-blind comparison of 22 commonly prescribed pediatric antibiotic suspensions rated some suspensions as unpalatable enough to jeopardize patient compliance with therapy. Among the suspensions suggested for second-line therapy for AOM that were judged very unpalatable, based on overall scores of 2 or lower on a scale of 1 (lowest) to 10 (highest) for appearance, smell, texture, taste, and aftertaste were cefuroxime, cefpodoxime, and erythromycin-sulfisoxazole.[31] The macrolide clarithromycin and the generic formulation of TMP/SMX have also been rated as having poor palatability.[22] Of interest, infants <6 months old appear to have poorly developed ability to taste bitter substances, so they may accept unpalatable drugs somewhat better than older children. Use of masking flavors added to each dose can also allow better compliance of unpalatable drugs. One can use chocolate syrup or a commercial product such as FLAVORx. The latter comes in 102 flavors and costs $4 to $5 for 50 doses.

Dosing Schedule and Administration

Adherence to a medication's recommended administration schedule improves if the antibiotic is given once a day (80% compliance) or at most twice a day (69% compliance). Dosing three times a day hampers compliance (38% compliance).[32] Antibiotic effectiveness in children is not altered if the drug is administered in the "fed" state (when food is in the stomach or small intestine). Infants and children often accept a dose of medication more willingly with a bottle or when juice or a snack is offered simultaneously with or just after the medication, particularly for clarithromycin, cefuroxime, and cefpodoxime. Amoxicillin/clavulanate should always be given with food or milk to decrease rates of diarrhea and gastritis. For children weighing >30 kg, clinicians have sometimes sprinkled the capsule formulation of cefdinir on applesauce to achieve a higher dose at a lower cost.

Duration of Therapy

Shorter-course therapy appears to occur often; despite instructions to the contrary, many patients stop taking a prescribed antibiotic when symptoms abate. Many β-lactam antibiotics are equally effective with a shorter course while improving compliance and reducing cost.

The results of numerous trials of shorter (2- to 7-day) courses of β-lactam antibiotic therapy for AOM show that an adequate course of therapy depends on the child's age and severity of AOM:

- Along with azithromycin, both cefpodoxime and cefdinir are approved for 5-day AOM therapy
- Azithromycin is FDA approved for 3-day and single-dose AOM therapy.[33]
- A not-yet-approved formulation of azithromycin (20 mg/kg/day for 3 days) has undergone clinical testing and was compared with high-dose amoxicillin/clavulanate in a single tympanocentesis trial. The double dose of azithromycin for 3 days was equivalent in clinical outcome at end of therapy. However, this was an international study, which had a low recovery rate of pathogens (55%) and a much lower rate of resistant pathogens than is seen customarily in US studies using tympanocentesis.[34]
- For children >2 years old with uncomplicated AOM (no otorrhea, no concurrent illness, no

119

persistent/refractory/recurrent AOM), 5 to 7 days of β-lactam antibiotic therapy may be adequate and may reflect the caregiver's actual medication administration practice[35] (the American Academy of Pediatrics [AAP]/American Academy of Family Physicians [AAFP] guideline suggests after age 5 years[36])

- Short-course therapy (5 days) with amoxicillin/clavulanate was statistically less effective than 10 days of therapy in children <2 years of age.[37] Short-course therapy even with highly efficacious drugs may fail in difficult-to-treat populations, such as younger children.

- However, the full 10-day course of β-lactam antibiotic medication improves efficacy rates in children:
  - With refractory AOM[38]
  - Younger than 24 months
  - With severe or complicated AOM (eg, perforation of the tympanic membrane [TM])
  - At higher risk for treatment failure (eg, due to underlying medical conditions)
  - Who are otitis prone.

■ Nontreatment of AOM in Young Children
AAP/AAFP Guideline

For the group of children who have a "certain" diagnosis of AOM, the observation option or "masterful inactivity" is a consideration for only a select group according to the AAP/AAFP guideline, ie, only in children >24 months who have fever <39°C and mild or no otalgia. For children who have an "uncertain" diagnosis of AOM, the observation option can be considered for the child age 6 to 24 months if the child's symptomatology is considered nonsevere. For the child >24 months old with an "uncertain" diagnosis, the observation *option* is considered as a possible standard of care.

The AAP/AAFP guideline does not recommend the observation option for children younger than 24 months who have a "certain" diagnosis of AOM (**Table 6.6**). Damoiseaux and colleagues[39] compared amoxicillin therapy with placebo in 240 Dutch children ages 6- to 24-months old. The study was conducted by 53 general practitioners (~5 patients per MD); one third of the originally enrolled children were lost to follow-up.

In the 117 amoxicillin-treated children and the 123 placebo-treated children, persistent symptoms (fever, earache, irritability, crying) were noted at day 4 in 65% and 72%, respectively. Furthermore, clinical failure at day 11 was observed in 64% and 70%, respectively, a much higher failure rate than has been reported in the United States. These data clearly show that for children younger than 24 months, most will have significant persistent symptoms at both 4 days and 11 days, an outcome unacceptable for any practitioner. Of particular concern is the fact that four patients in the placebo-

TABLE 6.6 — 2004 AAP/AAFP AOM Guidelines: Who to Treat		
Age	**Certain Diagnosis**	**Uncertain Diagnosis**
<6 mo	Antibiotics	Antibiotics
6 mo to 2 y	Antibiotics	Antibiotics; may consider observation if nonsevere
>2 y	Antibiotics; observe if nonsevere	May consider observation
Abbreviations: AAFP, American Academy of Family Physicians; AAP, American Academy of Pediatrics; AOM, acute otitis media.		
Severe = moderate to severe otalgia, fever >39°C. Observe only if follow-up is adequate and caregiver agrees; give antibiotics if symptoms worsen or persist.		
Modified from: AAP/AAFP. *Pediatrics*. 2004;113:1451-1465.		

treated group were hospitalized for AOM, dehydration, and meningitis, and one for unspecified reasons.[40]

Use of placebo therapy theoretically relies on natural defenses, which are usually effective by 7 days in 80% to 90% of children >2 years old who are not otitis prone. However, febrile children with otalgia in the United States appear nearly 3-fold more likely to have *S pneumoniae* as the pathogen.[41] This pathogen also spontaneously resolves in only ~20% of children by 3 to 6 days and therefore these children may be at increased risk for bacteremia or other complications if no therapy is used. However, with universal use of PCV-7, the risk of such invasive disease is dramatically reduced. Therefore, the watchful waiting option for AOM may be less risky for children who have received at least three doses of PCV-7. Nonetheless, some experts disagree with the nontreatment option at any age.

The nontreatment recommendation is based primarily on the meta-analysis from Rosenfeld's review of nine randomized controlled clinical trials using nontreatment performed between 1968 and 2000.[42]

■ Our Perspective Regarding Nontreatment Option

One prominent pediatric infectious disease expert disagrees with the nontreatment option based on the following reasons[43,44]:

- Children <2 years of age were excluded from three of the nine studies in the meta-analysis.
- Mean age of study children was 4 years, thus a minority of children were <2 years old in whom AOM is the most difficult to treat.
- Two investigations excluded all children in whom antibiotics were thought to be indicated.
- Diagnoses of AOM were based on TM findings of MEE plus the presence of symptoms, but they did not differentiate between AOM and

OME. OME is clearly a disease that is mostly nonbacterial and would almost never respond to antibiotics.

- Children were not a random sample and often excluded those with more severe symptoms which would bias the results in the direction of no difference.
- In five of nine studies, an inappropriate antibiotic (penicillin V) or insufficient dose of the antimicrobial was used.
- Despite these inadequacies, six of the studies still showed antibiotic superiority over placebo.

Another recent study evaluating children who had acute tympanostomy tube otorrhea compared amoxicillin/clavulanate with placebo. An almost 2-fold higher clinical cure rate was observed in children treated with amoxicillin/clavulanate vs those who were observed (82% vs 40%).[44]

McCormick and colleagues studied 223 patients, ages 6 months to 12 years (57% younger than 24 months), who were 73% nonwhite and 83% not fully vaccinated with PCV-7, comparing high-dose amoxicillin with nontreatment for AOM.[45] One third of patients in the watchful-waiting group required antibiotic intervention for worsening AOM, and the antibiotic-treatment group experienced 16% fewer failures. However, parental satisfaction was comparable between both groups at end of therapy.

The study was limited by the use of minimal criteria in AOM symptom scores and in otoscopic scores for AOM diagnosis. Otitis symptom scores ≥4 included children who had some form of one or all of the following three symptoms: ear pain, irritability, or decreased activity, based on a scale of 1 (no symptoms) to 7 (severe symptoms). This study obviously included many children who had minimal symptoms. Since the scores could range from 3 to 21, the average score was about 8 (mild symptoms); only a score of ≥4 was required for inclusion.

An otoscopic score was based on a scale of 0 to 7. A score between 3 and 5 included children who had erythema or opacification, but none had bulging of the TM. Children with these criteria accounted for 78% and 70% of patients in amoxicillin- and watchful-waiting groups, respectively. In fact, 38% and 33%, respectively, merely had TMs with redness and, at most, a purulent air-fluid level. Thus most of the children had mild to marginal AOM.

In the watchful-waiting group, one half of patients were >2 years of age — a group in which spontaneous resolution, especially with mild AOM or OME, would be expected to occur more readily. The failure rate for children in the watchful-waiting group who had recently received antibiotics was also 52%. These data on watchful waiting, although limited by the small sample size and the predominance of minimal AOM, do suggest that watchful waiting may be considered for older children who have mild AOM and in whom very careful followup can be assured. However, all these notable limitations also preclude using these data to make any changes in the AAP/AAFP guidelines on AOM about the use of watchful waiting for children <2 years of age with AOM.

Until the medical community is more comfortable with nontreatment of AOM,[46] practitioners cautiously could introduce the idea into their practices under the following conditions:

- Questionable or uncertain diagnosis of AOM
- Child is >2 years old
- Episode of AOM occurs >3 months since the previous episode
- Asymptomatic AOM
- Fever <100.8°F
- Parents who concur with no therapy.

It may be reasonable to have an informed consent document about risks and benefits of nontreatment which has been discussed, signed, and placed on the chart. Possible risks would include chronic hearing loss, meningitis, mastoiditis, subdural venous thrombosis, otitic hydrocephalus, cholesteatoma—many of which would sometimes occur whether the case of bona fide AOM was treated or not (see Chapter 10, *Complications*).[47]

If practitioners follow the AAP/AAFP guideline, we are concerned that many clinicians who are too busy, too inexperienced, or too pressured will dispense antibiotic prescriptions for any child under 6 months and for those who have more fever or generic symptoms from 6 to 24 months of age when the TMs have not been examined. In children <24 months of age, the category of "uncertain" AOM diagnosis will almost certainly lower the standard for stringency and diligence to diagnose AOM for clinicians who are less than thorough or who use inadequate equipment. As long as one alleges diagnostic uncertainty for the TM in a cranky or febrile child (as shown in **Table 6.6**), this algorithm now apparently sanctions antibiotic treatment for any child younger than 6 months or for a more symptomatic child 6 to 24 months old.

In young children, ear canals and TMs are particularly difficult to clean and assess, respectively. Imagine the tremendous ease and appeal of the "uncertain" diagnosis in a sick youngster during hectic epidemics of respiratory syncytial virus, influenza, adenovirus, etc. Refractory cerumen can usually be removed via gentle lavage with a water irrigation device (eg, the Water-Pik TM at low setting) as long as a ventilating tube or otorrhea is not present. If the TM cannot be visualized due to cerumen or traumatic cleaning, another diligent effort should be made within 24 to 48 hours, particularly before escalating up the antibiotic scale due to persistent symptoms. Use of softening agents (eg, Debrox drops) for several days prior to a return visit can be useful as well. Otherwise, otolaryngology referral may be in order, especially before embarking upon multiple courses of broad-spectrum antibiotics without a real diagnosis.

Note that high-dose amoxicillin/clavulanate is the designated initial antibiotic choice for a "severe" and "uncertain" diagnosis. Two days later, if fever or irritability persists from the viral infection, parenteral ceftriaxone for 3 days is the recommended choice, even though AOM has still not been assured.

Algorithm for Selection of Antibiotic Therapy for AOM

Based on efficacy, the overall prevalence of antibiotic-resistant AOM pathogens in PCV-7–vaccinated children, potential for adverse effects, and patient compliance issues (less serious side effects, cost, palatability, and dosing schedule), we developed the algorithm shown in **Figure 6.4** for management of AOM diagnosed by strict criteria in an otherwise healthy child between 6 and 36 months old. Subsequent chapters detail the rationale for antibiotic choices for each level of therapy. An algorithm for the treatment of the penicillin-allergic child with AOM is shown in **Figure 7.3**.

Additional Considerations in Antibiotic Therapy for AOM

Additional considerations in the use of antibiotic therapy for AOM are the management of otorrhea, follow-up care, the role of viruses in AOM, the "Pollyanna effect" in judging the success of antibiotic therapy in treating AOM, and antibiotic overprescribing.

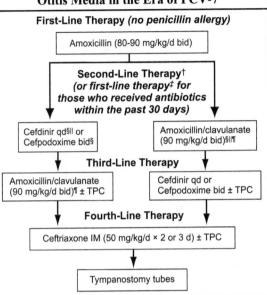

FIGURE 6.4 — Antibiotic Choices for Acute Otitis Media in the Era of PCV-7*

First-Line Therapy *(no penicillin allergy)*

Amoxicillin (80-90 mg/kg/d bid)

**Second-Line Therapy†
(or first-line therapy‡ for
those who received antibiotics
within the past 30 days)**

Cefdinir qd§‖ or
Cefpodoxime bid§

Amoxicillin/clavulanate
(90 mg/kg/d bid)§‖¶

Third-Line Therapy

Amoxicillin/clavulanate
(90 mg/kg/d bid)¶ ± TPC

Cefdinir qd or
Cefpodoxime bid ± TPC

Fourth-Line Therapy

Ceftriaxone IM (50 mg/kg/d × 2 or 3 d) ± TPC

Tympanostomy tubes

Abbreviation: AOM, acute otitis media; IM, intramuscularly; TPC, tympanocentesis with culture and susceptibility testing.

* Recommendations are for children 6 to 36 months old with AOM. In the opinion of the authors, this algorithm will apply to children as young as 3 months old.

† If fully vaccinated with pneumococcal conjugated heptavalent vaccine, although controversial, cefixime might be considered as an option by some experts. Its use for AOM is limited by its minimal coverage of penicillin-susceptible *Streptococcus pneumoniae* (PSSP) and lack of coverage for penicillin-nonsusceptible *S pneumoniae* (PNSP).

‡ Azithromycin (1, 3, or 5 days) may be an alternative for the older child with recurrent AOM who has 1) concomitant pneumonia suggestive of atypical pathogens, 2) significant acute gastroenteritis. Azithromycin's coverage of *Haemophilus influenzae* is limited (~50%), in double tympanocentesis studies at the mid-therapy visit. To improve *H influenzae* coverage, some experts add trimethoprim/sulfamethoxazole to azithromycin, resulting in an off-label combination of two FDA-approved AOM drugs.

§ Children coinfected with AOM and acute conjunctivitis should be treated with a combination of eye drops (trimethoprim sulfate and polymyxin B sulphate or topical fluoroquinolone) and an oral antibiotic for AOM which covers β-lactamase (+) *H influenzae* because of the high prevalence of *H influenzae* in these cases. These antibiotics would include cefdinir, cefpodoxime, and amoxicillin/clavulanate.

‖ If coinfected with impetigo and AOM, cefdinir and amoxicillin/clavulanate can be started empirically to cover both AOM and impetigo.

¶ Augmentin ES-600: formulation is amoxicillin 600 mg + clavulanate 6.4 mg/5 mL.

■ Management of Otorrhea

Children with suspected otorrhea (purulent fluid draining from a perforated TM or intact tympanostomy tube) should be examined within 24 hours of onset, and if otorrhea is documented, an oral antibiotic should be started. In some cases, cerumen draining from the ear canal may be mistaken for otorrhea.

If the child has otorrhea through a spontaneously perforated TM and no additional risk factors, antibiotic choices are the same as if the TM were intact (**Figure 6.4**). Topical antibiotics are not indicated. However, if the child has otorrhea with a tympanostomy tube, for children vaccinated with PCV-7, data indirectly suggest that the risk of PNSP is probably low.[5] Bacterial cultures of acute tube otorrhea are not usually performed. Bacterial cultures of tube otorrhea in the first 48 hours of drainage are positive for an otopathogen in only about one third of cases but are reasonably accurate in predicting the middle ear pathogen. After 48 hours, cultures usually reveal external ear flora that expand in numbers after the canal becomes full of wet, proteinaceous drainage. At this point *Pseudomonas*, *Enterobacter*, *Staphylococcus* species, or *Proteus* will predominate. After 48 hours, more reliable cultures may be obtained by cleaning/suctioning the external canal under direct vision and obtaining a direct culture from the pressure-equalizing (PE) tube orifice.

Children without PE tubes who develop otorrhea should be seen at the end of therapy to determine whether there are persisting low levels of drainage, whether a perforation has developed, and that a cholesteatoma is not present. Cholesteatoma (see Chapter 9, *Tympanostomy Tubes*) is one of the rare complications of AOM and previous tubes, and often presents with malodorous otorrhea.

When no fever or otalgia is present, otorrhea through PE tubes can often be managed with topical therapy (Ciprodex [ciprofloxacin plus dexamethasone] or Floxin [ofloxacin] otic drops) for 7 to 14 days, plus keeping the canal free from external water contamination. Ciprodex and Floxin are the only drugs indicated by the Food and Drug Administration for acute tube otorrhea. A recent clinical trial compared Ciprodex vs Floxin in children with acute tube otorrhea. This study reported that the combination Ciprodex was superior to Floxin for clinical cure (90% vs 78%) and microbiologic success (92% vs 82%), and resulted in a shorter median time to cessation of otorrhea (4 days vs 6 days).

Roland and colleagues studied ciprofloxacin/dexamethasone vs topical ciprofloxacin alone in 201 children aged 6 months to 12 years with AOM with tympanostomy tubes of ≤3 weeks' duration and visible otorrhea. The mean time to cessation of otorrhea was significantly shorter with topical ciprofloxacin/dexamethasone than with ciprofloxacin alone — a 20% reduction in time to cessation of otorrhea.[48]

Many experts have concerns that the topical aminoglycosides (tobramycin, gentamicin, neomycin) may be ototoxic; thus we do not recommend them.[49] They also are minimally less expensive, even in generic formulations, and they provide less coverage for otopathogens.[50]

■ Follow-Up Care

Figure 6.5 shows a suggested schedule for follow-up care after outpatient treatment of an episode of AOM in a young child.

Every routine pediatric office visit for illness or a checkup should include an evaluation for MEE by pneumatic otoscopy. Confirmation by use of tympanometry may be considered to corroborate OME when clinicians are uncertain. Antibiotics are not recommended nor are they useful to treat OME (see AAP guideline section on the diagnosis of AOM). If behav-

FIGURE 6.5 — Follow-Up Schedule After Outpatient Treatment for an Episode of Acute Otitis Media in a Young Child

Day 0—Caregiver should be instructed to contact the office or clinic if:
- Earache persists
- Other signs of infection persist or worsen
- Caregiver suspects that treatment is causing new problem

Day 2—Follow-up visit should be scheduled on day 2 of antibiotic therapy if the child:
- Has severe systemic symptoms initially
- Is immunocompromised

Days 10-14—A follow-up visit is indicated only for children:
- Who are otitis prone
- Who had otorrhea
- Who have failed several courses of antibiotics
- In whom acute otitis media symptoms recur

6 Weeks—Follow-up visit is desirable to determine whether middle ear effusion has resolved if no routine checkup is normally scheduled within 1 to 3 months in children <36 months old

ior problems, speech difficulties, or school performance problems arise, PE tubes may be considered.

■ Viruses in AOM

As noted in Chapter 3, *Pathophysiology, Immunology, and Natural History*, a viral upper respiratory infection (URI) usually precedes and predisposes to AOM. Although viruses are rarely (5% to 6%) the only pathogens isolated from the MEE of a child with AOM, they produce inflammatory mediators. The presence of viruses in the middle ear is often predictive of a higher antibiotic failure rate.[51]

In support of this hypothesis, in the United States, Canafax and colleagues found that amoxicillin penetration into the MEE was reduced in children with viral infection. From this finding, they concluded that traditional amoxicillin dosing recommendation of 40 mg/kg/d in three divided doses was inadequate to effectively eradicate PNSP, particularly during viral co-infection. Therefore, they recommended dosing amoxicillin at 75 to 90 mg/kg/d for AOM,[52] as have others.[53,54]

On the other hand, Pitkaranta and colleagues (in Finland) found no important differences in the risk of treatment failure, relapse, or recurrence of AOM between children with and those without virus in the MEE.[55]

■ Antibiotic Overprescription

Antibacterial drugs are not effective in treating viral infections. Nevertheless, clinicians are under great pressure to prescribe these drugs for children with an illness. The magnitude of this practice of antibiotic overprescription in the United States is evident from a report that about 60% of patients in the Kentucky Medicaid database with a diagnosis of the common cold were treated with antibiotics.[56]

In many studies, particularly those conducted previously in Europe, the diagnosis of AOM did not include documentation of MEE and did not exclude symptoms such as fever and irritability attributable to viral URI.[39,57,58] Although AOM is a sequela in one fourth to one half of viral URIs in children,[59] AOM should not be diagnosed based on symptoms alone. We also think that the diagnosis of AOM should be a visual one (see Chapter 4, *Diagnosis*) and that the presence of nonpurulent MEE plus symptoms is not indicative of AOM.

In this age of escalating antibiotic resistance, clinicians need to keep the following adage in mind: Treating nonbacterial (eg, viral) infections such as bronchitis, colds, bronchiolitis, or OME with antibiotics is futile, expensive, and promotes antibiotic resistance.[35] Ideally, education of parents about the consequences of improper use of antibiotics is preferred. Important educational points include:

- Low but definite risk of adverse reaction and allergy
- Increased expense
- Promotion of bacterial resistance.[60]

In a study by Palmer and colleagues, 300 parents from a suburban private practice and 100 parents from the inner city were surveyed for antibiotic use patterns. The authors found that 18% of parents gave antibiotics prior to office visit, 14% say they should have received an antibiotic when none was given at an office visit, and 9% said that the antibiotic was not necessary.[61]

In a study evaluating prescribing practices of pediatricians in Memphis, Tennessee, the authors observed the following:

- 81% of children received an antibiotic at each office visit
- 59% of these prescriptions were not for AOM

- Nearly all prescriptions were for broad-spectrum cephalosporins.[62,63]

In a study surveying 61 pediatricians in Massachusetts, the authors found that:
- 71% felt parents demanded an unnecessary antibiotic more than four times per month and 35% acquiesced and gave the antibiotic prescription to the family
- 61% said patients wanted a different antibiotic from the one they wanted to prescribe at least four times in the previous month
- One third prescribed an antibiotic when it was not indicated
- 19% occasionally phoned in an antibiotic.[64]

REFERENCES

1. Block SL. Management of acute otitis media in the 1990s. The decade of resistant pneumococcus. *Paediatr Drugs*. 1999;1:31-50.

2. Eskola J, Kilpi T, Palmu A, et al. Efficacy of a pneumococcal conjugate vaccine against acute otitis media. *N Engl J Med*. 2001;344:403-409.

3. Block SL, Hedrick J, Harrison CJ, et al. Community-wide vaccination with the heptavalent pneumococcal conjugate significantly alters the microbiology of acute otitis media. *Pediatr Infect Dis J*. 2004;23:829-833.

4. Casey JR, Pichichero ME. Changes in frequency and pathogens causing acute otitis media in 1995-2003. *Pediatr Infect Dis J*. 2004;23:824-828.

5. Caspary H, Welch JC, Lawson L, et al. Impact of pneumococcal polysaccharide vaccine (Prevnar) on middle ear fluid in children undergoing tympanostomy tube insertion. *Laryngoscope*. 2004;114:975-980.

6. Sutton DV, Derkay CS, Darrow DH, Strasnick B. Resistant bacteria in middle ear fluid at the time of tympanostomy tube surgery. *Ann Otol Rhinol Laryngol.* 2000;109:24-29.

7. McEllistrem MC, Adams J, Mason EO, Wald ER. Epidemiology of acute otitis media caused by *Streptococcus pneumoniae* before and after licensure of the 7-valent pneumococcal protein conjugate vaccine. *J Infect Dis.* 2003;188:1679-1684.

8. Samore MH, Magill MK, Alder SC, et al. High rates of multiple antibiotic resistance in *Streptococcus pneumoniae* from healthy children living in isolated rural communities: association with cephalosporin use and intrafamilial transmission. *Pediatrics.* 2001;108:856-865.

9. Eldan M, Leibovitz E, Piglansky L, et al. Predictive value of pneumococcal nasopharyngeal cultures for the assessment of nonresponsive acute otitis media in children. *Pediatr Infect Dis J.* 2000;19:298-303.

10. Pelton SI, Loughlin AM, Marchant CD. Seven valent pneumococcal conjugate vaccine immunization in two Boston communities: changes in serotypes and antimicrobial susceptibility among *Streptococcus pneumoniae* isolates. *Pediatr Infect Dis J.* 2004;23:1015-1022.

11. Neu HC. Otitis media: antibiotic resistance of causative pathogens and treatment alternatives. *Pediatr Infect Dis J.* 1995;14:S51-S56.

12. *Physicians' Desk Reference.* 59th ed. Montvale, NJ: Medical Economics Company; 2005.

13. Marchant CD, Carlin SA, Johnson CE, Shurin PA. Measuring the comparative efficacy of antibacterial agents for acute otitis media: the "Pollyanna phenomenon." *J Pediatr.* 1992;120:72-77.

14. Carlin SA, Marchant CD, Shurin PA, Johnson CE, Super DM, Rehmus JM. Host factors and early therapeutic response in acute otitis media. *J Pediatr.* 1991;118:178-183.

15. Rodriguez WJ, Schwartz RH, Thorne MM. Increasing incidence of penicillin- and ampicillin-resistant middle ear pathogens. *Pediatr Infect Dis J*. 1995;14:1075-1078.

16. Block SL, Harrison CJ, Hedrick JA, et al. Penicillin-resistant *Streptococcus pneumoniae* in acute otitis media: risk factors, susceptibility patterns and antimicrobial management. *Pediatr Infect Dis J*. 1995;14:751-759.

17. Block SL, Hedrick JA, Harrison CJ, et al. Increasing rates of resistance in acute otitis media [Abstract 53]. Abstracts of the 39th Interscience Conference on Antimicrobial Agents and Chemotherapy, September 1999, San Francisco, Calif. Washington, DC: American Society for Microbiology, 2000.

18. Block SL, Hedrick JA, Smith RA, et al. Pathogens of acute otitis media (AOM) in a pediatric population [Abstract K23]. Abstracts of the 36th Interscience Conference on Antimicrobial Agents and Chemotherapy; September 1996; New Orleans, La. Washington, DC: American Society for Microbiology; 1996:253.

19. Block SL, Hammerschlag MR, Hedrick J, et al. *Chlamydia pneumoniae* in acute otitis media. *Pediatr Infect Dis J*. 1997; 16:858-862.

20. Harrison CJ, Marks MI, Welch DF. Microbiology of recently treated acute otitis media compared with previously untreated acute otitis media. *Pediatr Infect Dis J*. 1985;4:641-646.

21. Del Beccaro MA, Mendelman PM, Inglis AF, et al. Bacteriology of acute otitis media: a new perspective. *J Pediatr*. 1992;120:81-84.

22. Pichichero ME. Empiric antibiotic selection criteria for respiratory infections in pediatric practice. *Pediatr Infect Dis J*. 1997;16(suppl 3):S60-S64.

23. Blumer JL. Fundamental basis for rational therapeutics in acute otitis media. *Pediatr Infect Dis J*. 1999;18:1130-1140.

24. Jacobs MR, Bajaksouzian S, Zilles A, Lin G, Pankuch GA, Appelbaum PC. Susceptibilities of *Streptococcus pneumoniae* and *Haemophilus influenzae* to 10 oral antimicrobial agents based on pharmacodynamic parameters: 1997 U.S. Surveillance Study. *Antimicrob Agents Chemother.* 1999;43:1901-1908.

25. Thornsberry C, Ogilvie PT, Holley HP Jr, Sahm DF. Survey of susceptibilities of *Streptococcus pneumoniae, Haemophilus influenzae,* and *Moraxella catarrhalis* isolates to 26 antimicrobial agents: a prospective U.S. study. *Antimicrob Agents Chemother.* 1999;43:2612-2623.

26. Jacobs MR, Dagan R, Appelbaum PC, Burch DJ. Prevalence of antimicrobial-resistant pathogens in middle ear fluid: multinational study of 917 children with acute otitis media. *Antimicrob Agents Chemother.* 1998;42:589-595.

27. Sader HS, Fritsche TR, Mutnick AH, Jones RN. Contemporary evaluation of the in vitro activity and spectrum of cefdinir compared with other orally administered antimicrobials tested against common respiratory tract pathogens (2000-2002). *Diagn Microbiol Infect Dis.* 2003;47:515-525.

28. Boken DJ, Chartrand SA, Goering RV, Kruger R, Harrison CJ. Colonization with penicillin-resistant *Streptococcus pneumoniae* in a child-care center. *Pediatr Infect Dis J.* 1995;14:879-884.

29. Poole MD. Otitis media complications and treatment failures: implications of pneumococcal resistance. *Pediatr Infect Dis J.* 1995;14(suppl 4):S23-S26.

30. Whitney CG, Farley MM, Hadler J, et al, for the Active Bacterial Core Surveillance of the Emerging Infections Program Network. Decline in invasive pneumococcal disease after the introduction of protein-polysaccharide conjugate vaccine. *N Engl J Med.* 2003;348:1737-1746.

31. Steele RW, Thomas MP, Begue RE, et al. Selection of pediatric antibiotic suspensions: taste and cost factors. *Infect Med.* 1999;16:197-200.

32. Sclar DA, Tartaglione TA, Fine MJ. Overview of issues related to medical compliance with implications for the outpatient management of infectious diseases. *Infect Agents Dis.* 1994;3:266-273.

33. Block SL, Arrieta A, Seibel M, McLinn S, Eppes S, Murphy MJ. Single-dose (30 mg/kg) azithromycin compared with 10-day amoxicillin/clavulanate for the treatment of uncomplicated acute otitis media: a double-blind, placebo-controlled, randomized clinical trial. *Curr Ther Res Clin Exp.* 2003;64(suppl a):A30-A42.

34. Arrieta A, Arguedas A, Fernandez P, et al. High-dose azithromycin versus high-dose amoxicillin-clavulanate for treatment of children with recurrent or persistent acute otitis media. *Antimicrob Agents Chemother.* 2003;47:3179-3186.

35. Dowell SF, Marcy SM, Phillips WR, Gerber MA, Schwartz B. Otitis media-principles of judicious use of antimicrobial agents. *Pediatrics.* 1998;101(suppl):165-171.

36. American Academy of Pediatrics Subcommittee on Management of Acute Otitis Media. Diagnosis and management of acute otitis media. *Pediatrics.* 2004;113:1451-1465.

37. Hoberman A, Paradise JL, Burch DJ, et al. Equivalent efficacy and reduced occurrence of diarrhea from a new formulation of amoxicillin/clavulanate potassium (Augmentin) for treatmetn of acute otitis media in children. *Pediatr Infect Dis J.* 1997;16:463-470.

38. Paradise JL. Managing otitis media: a time for change. *Pediatrics.* 1995;96:712-715.

39. Damoiseaux RA, van Balen FA, Hoes AW, Verheij TJ, de Melker RA. Primary care based randomised, double blind trial of amoxicillin versus placebo for acute otitis media in children aged under 2 years. *BMJ.* 2000;320:350-354.

40. Rodriguez WJ, Schwartz RH. *Streptococcus pneumoniae* causes otitis media with higher fever and more redness of tympanic membranes than *Haemophilus influenzae* or *Moraxella catarrhalis. Pediatr Infect Dis J.* 1999;18:942-944.

6

41. Rosenfeld RM, Bluestone CD. *Evidence-Based Otitis Media*. 2nd ed. Hamilton, Canada: BC Decker; 2003.

42. Wald ER. Acute otitis media: more trouble with the evidence. *Pediatr Infect Dis J*. 2003;22:103-104.

43. Wald ER. To treat or not to treat. *Pediatrics*. 2005;115:1087-1089.

44. Ruohola A, Heikkinen T, Meurman O, Puhakka T, Lindblad N, Ruuskanen O. Antibiotic treatment of acute otorrhea through tympanostomy tube: randomized double-blind placebo-controlled study with daily follow-up. *Pediatrics*. 2003;111:1061-1067.

45. McCormick DP, Chonmaitree T, Pittman C, et al. Nonsevere acute otitis media: a clinical trial comparing outcomes of watchful waiting versus immediate antibiotic treatment. *Pediatrics*. 2005;115:1455-1465.

46. Finkelstein JA, Stille CJ, Rifas-Shiman SL, Goldmann D. Watchful waiting for acute otitis media: are parents and physicians ready? *Pediatrics*. 2005;115:1466-1473.

47. Go C, Bernstein JM, de Jong AL, Sulek M, Friedman EM. Intracranial complications of acute mastoiditis. *Int J Pediatr Otorhinolaryngol*. 2000;52:143-148.

48. Roland PS, Anon JB, Moe RD, et al. Topical ciprofloxacin/dexamethasone is superior to ciprofloxacin alone in pediatric patients with acute otitis media and otorrhea through tympanostomy tubes. *Laryngoscope*. 2003;113:2116-2122.

49. Roland PS, Kreisler LS, Reese B, et al. Topical ciprofloxacin/dexamethasone otic suspension is superior to ofloxacin otis solution in the treatment of children with acute otitis media with otorrhea through tympanostomy tubes. *Pediatrics*. 2004;113:e40-e46.

50. Block SL, Hedrick J, Tyler R, et al. Increasing bacterial resistance in pediatric acute conjunctivitis (1997-1998). *Antimicrob Agents Chemother*. 2000;44:1650-1654.

51. Ramilo O. Role of respiratory viruses in acute otitis media: implications for management. *Pediatr Infect Dis J.* 1999;18:1125-1129.

52. Canafax DM, Yuan Z, Chonmaitree T, Deka K, Russlie HQ, Giebink GS. Amoxicillin middle ear fluid penetration and pharmacokinetics in children with acute otitis media. *Pediatr Infect Dis J.* 1998;17:149-156.

53. Harrison CJ, Welch DF. Middle ear effusion amoxicillin concentrations in acute otitis media. *Pediatr Infect Dis J.* 1998;17:657-658.

54. Seikel K, Shelton S, McCracken GH. Middle ear fluid concentrations of amoxicillin after large dosages in children with acute otitis media. *Pediatr Infect Dis J.* 1997;16:710-711.

55. Pitkaranta A, Virolainen A, Jero J, Arruda E, Hayden FG. Detection of rhinovirus, respiratory syncytial virus, and coronavirus infections in acute otitis media by reverse transcriptase polymerase chain reaction. *Pediatrics.* 1998;102: 291-295.

56. Mainous AG, Hueston WJ, Clark JR. Antibiotics and upper respiratory infection: do some folks think there is a cure for the common cold? *J Fam Pract.* 1996;42:357-361.

57. Culpepper L, Froom J. Routine antimicrobial treatment of acute otitis media. Is it necessary? *JAMA.* 1997;278:1643-1645.

58. Del Mar C, Glasziou P, Hayem M. Are antibiotics indicated as initial treatment for children with acute otitis media? A meta-analysis. *BMJ.* 1997;314:1526-1529.

59. Heikkinen T. Temporal development of acute otitis media during upper respiratory tract infection. *Pediatr Infect Dis J.* 1994;13:659-661.

60. Werk LN, Bauchner H. Practical considerations when treating children with antimicrobials in the outpatient setting. *Drugs.* 1998;55:779-790.

6

61. Palmer DA, Bauchner H. Parents' and physicians' views on antibiotics. *Pediatrics*. 1997;99:E6.

62. Arnold KE, Leggiadro RJ, Breiman RF, et al. Risk factors for carriage of drug-resistant *Streptococcus pneumoniae* among children in Memphis, Tennessee. *J Pediatr*. 1996;128:757-764.

63. Edwards KM. Resisting the urge to prescribe. *J Pediatr*. 1996;128:729-730.

64. Bauchner H, Pelton SI, Klein JO. Parents, physicians, and antibiotic use. *Pediatrics*. 1999;103:395-401.

First-Line Antibiotic Therapy

First-line therapy with a narrow-spectrum, inexpensive agent is indicated for acute otitis media (AOM) patients at low risk for resistant pathogens (**Table 7.1**). As the algorithm in **Figure 6.4** shows, the first-line therapy for an episode of AOM in an otherwise healthy child (not penicillin allergic) between 4 and 36 months old and who has not received antibiotics in the past 30 days is amoxicillin (80-90 mg/kg/d) in two divided doses for 10 days. In light of data from Casey and Pichichero[1] and Block and colleagues,[2] if antibiotics have been received in the past 30 days, initial therapy for AOM should include a β-lactamase–stable drug. Their data suggest that almost half the pathogens in recurrent AOM are likely to be β-lactamase–producing gram-negative organisms. In essence, this shifts initial therapy in recent antibiotic recipients to the drugs listed as second-line therapy in **Figure 6.4**.

Before pneumococcal conjugate vaccine (PCV)–7, children <2 years of age and in day care had a higher risk of penicillin-nonsusceptible *Streptococcus pneumoniae* (PNSP), therefore, high-dose amoxicillin (90 mg/kg/d divided bid) was preferred in this population. Because we have no data on new-onset AOM in PCV-7 children and because the American Academy of Pediatrics and American Academy of Family Physician (AAP/AAFP) guideline recommends high-dose amoxicillin,[3] we still believe that high-dose amoxicillin should be the preferred initial therapy for uncomplicated AOM. However, Garbutt and colleagues differ with this opinion.[4] In the St. Louis area, the prevalence of PNSP in the nasopharynx of symptomatic children

TABLE 7.1 — Risks of Contracting Resistant Acute Otitis Media Pathogen

Condition	Low Risk	High Risk	Degree of Risk
Recent acute otitis media	>1 month	<1 month	Major
Previous antibiotic use	>1 month	<1 month	Major
Day care attendance	No	Yes	Moderate
Sibling with resistant pathogen	No	Yes	Moderate
Less than 2 years of age	No	Yes	Minor
Seasonal (December to May)	No	Yes	Minor

The presence of either major risk factor or a combination of either moderate risk factor with both minor risk factors indicates a need for second-line therapy (Centers for Disease Control [CDC] recommendation).

was <5%. Therefore, these authors believe that children who have uncomplicated AOM should be treated with standard-dose amoxicillin. They still advocate high-dose amoxicillin for children attending day care or children with recurrent AOM.

AAP/AAFP Guideline

The AAP/AAFP guideline allows only three exceptions to the rule of using amoxicillin as first-line therapy (**Table 7.2** and **Table 7.3**)[3]:

- Penicillin allergy
- Febrile AOM
- Moderate to severe otalgia.

For the child who has febrile AOM or who has moderate to severe otalgia, the guideline recommends amoxicillin/clavulanate as the antibiotic of choice. We have concerns about this antibiotic choice in these two scenarios.

The primary rationale behind using amoxicillin/clavulanate over amoxicillin alone in AOM is to add the clavulanic acid component to provide coverage for β-lactamase–producing organisms. Children who are febrile with AOM most commonly are coinfected with viruses, which are the likely source of their fever. Also in the febrile child, the primary concern for practitioners is the possibility of occult bacteremia due to *S pneumoniae*. Clavulanate adds no additional coverage for *S pneumoniae*. Also, no data in the United States support the fact that children with fever or moderate to severe otalgia will *uncommonly* have β-lactamase–producing organisms as a cause of their AOM. In fact, before PCV-7 data were available, *S pneumoniae* was 4-fold more commonly isolated in children with otalgia and fever than was a β-lactamase–producing organism.[5] Furthermore, children with fever or more severe otalgia tend to eat and drink poorly. This exac-

TABLE 7.2 — AAP/AAFP Recommended Antibacterial Agents for Patients Who Are Not Penicillin Allergic and Are Being Treated Initially With Antibacterial Agents or Have Failed 48 to 72 Hours of Observation or Initial Management With Antibacterial Agents

Temperature ≥39°C and/or Severe Otalgia	At Diagnosis for Patients Being Treated Initially With Antibacterial Agents: Recommended	Clinically Defined Treatment Failure at 48–72 Hours After Initial Management With Observation Option: Recommended	Clinically Defined Treatment Failure at 48–72 Hours After Initial Management With Antibacterial Agents: Recommended
No	Amoxicillin 80–90 mg/kg per day	Amoxicillin 80–90 mg/kg per day	Amoxicillin/clavulanate 90/6.4 mg/kg per day
Yes	Amoxicillin/clavulanate 90/6.4 mg/kg per day	Amoxicillin/clavulanate 90/6.4 mg/kg per day	Ceftriaxone, 3 days

Abbreviations: AAFP, American Academy of Family Physicians; AAP, American Academy of Pediatrics.

Modified from: AAP/AAFP. *Pediatrics.* 2004;113:1451-1465.

Temperature ≥39°C and/or Severe Otalgia	At Diagnosis for Patients Being Treated Initially With Antibacterial Agents: Alternative for Penicillin Allergy	Clinically Defined Treatment Failure at 48–72 Hours After Initial Management With Observation Option: Alternative for Penicillin Allergy	Clinically Defined Treatment Failure at 48–72 Hours After Initial Management With Antibacterial Agents: Alternative for Penicillin Allergy
No	Non-type 1: cefdinir, cefuroxime, cefpodoxime; type 1: azithromycin, clarithromycin	Non-type 1: cefdinir, cefuroxime, cefpodoxime; type 1: azithromycin, clarithromycin	Non-type 1: ceftriaxone, 3 days; type 1: clindaycin
Yes	Ceftriaxone, 1 or 3 days	Ceftriaxone, 1 or 3 days	Tympanocentesis, clindamycin

TABLE 7.3 — AAP/AAFP Recommended Antibacterial Agents for Patients Who Are Penicillin Allergic and Are Being Treated Initially With Antibacterial Agents or Have Failed 48 to 72 Hours of Observation or Initial Management With Antibacterial Agents

Abbreviations: AAFP, American Academy of Family Physicians; AAP, American Academy of Pediatrics.

Modified from: AAP/AAFP. *Pediatrics.* 2004;113:1451-1465.

7

erbates the likelihood of gastrointestinal (GI) distress and vomiting that commonly occur with amoxicillin/clavulanate ingestion. This could be especially precarious for the occasional incidence of a child who has an occult bacteremia. We think that amoxicillin should provide suitable coverage in either of these scenarios with its superior palatability and lack of significant risk for the GI distress compared with amoxicillin/clavulanate.

Our Perspective

The exceptions to the rule of using amoxicillin as first-line therapy include the following:

- Penicillin allergy
- Recurrent AOM (β-lactamase–stable drug needed)
- Coinfection:
  - Impetigo (*Staphylococcus aureus* coverage needed)
  - Purulent conjunctivitis (*Haemophilus influenzae* coverage needed)
  - Pneumonia (additional coverage for *Mycoplasma* and *Chlamydia pneumoniae* with macrolides may be desirable).

The presence of either major risk factors (**Table 7.1**) or combination of either moderate risk factor plus both minor risk factors indicates a need for second-line antibiotic choice (Centers for Disease Control [CDC] recommendation).

Rationale for Amoxicillin and Twice-Daily Dosing

Despite the wide prevalence of bacterial strains resistant to amoxicillin, it remains the first-line therapy for AOM in children because of its:

- Recommendation by the AAP/AAFP guideline
- "Gold standard" of efficacy against pneumococcal infection and the most potent inexpensive Food and Drug Administration–approved oral pneumococcal drug
- Proven safety in nonallergic patients
- Few and mild side effects
- Inexpensiveness
- Palatable suspension formulation
- Narrowest-spectrum antibiotic indicated for AOM, thus sparing broader-spectrum AOM antibiotics for more difficult to treat cases
- Also, many cases of AOM are overdiagnosed by clinicians, so its use will "spare" broader-spectrum antibiotics for those who really need them.

Administering the daily dose of amoxicillin in two rather than three doses is preferred because:

- Two larger doses may improve efficacy, based on pharmacokinetic and pharmacodynamic findings of:
  – Higher peak plasma drug concentration (maximum concentration [C_{max}])
  – Larger area under the (plasma concentration) curve (AUC) (**Figure 7.1**)
  – Longer time above minimum inhibitory concentration (MIC) (**Figure 7.1**).
- Twice-daily dosing elicits significantly better patient compliance.[6]

Rationale for High-Dose vs Standard-Dose Amoxicillin

The traditional daily dose of amoxicillin for AOM is currently 40 mg/kg/d. Some experts now recommend 80-90 mg/kg/d divided bid as the standard dose. The Drug-Resistant *Streptococcus pneumoniae* Therapeu-

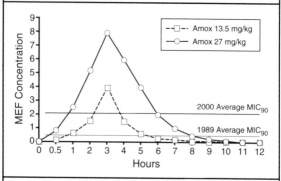

FIGURE 7.1 — Effect of Amoxicillin Dosing Change

To be effective, amoxicillin must exceed the MIC at least 40% of the time between doses, ie, 5 hours/dose on a bid schedule or 3.5 hours/dose on a tid schedule.

Abbreviations: MEF, middle ear fluid; MIC_{90}, minimum inhibitory concentration needed to inhibit growth [of pathogen] by 90%.

Harrison CJ, et al. *Pediatr Infect Dis J.* 1998;17:657-658.

tic Working Group, a consensus panel of the CDC,[7] and the AAP/AAFP[3] recommend high-dose amoxicillin (80-90 mg/kg/d) as first-line therapy in certain young children with AOM based on:

- The high prevalence of PNSP in AOM before PCV-7

- The safety and tolerability of amoxicillin at higher than standard doses (no significant increase in risk of side effects [eg, diarrhea] until dose exceeds 90 mg/kg/d)

- Evidence that higher doses of amoxicillin achieve concentrations in middle ear effusion (MEE) that may be sufficient to treat PNSP in AOM.[8-10] **Figure 7.2** shows that MEE concentrations with traditional-dose amoxicillin are usually <2 mg/mL but those with high-dose amoxicillin usually exceed the 2 mg/mL goal.[8]

- Up to 10% to 20% of children taking standard doses (~13 mg/kg) of amoxicillin have no detectable amoxicillin in MEE, while at 30 mg/kg/dose, all will have at least 1 mg/mL[8,10,11] (**Figure 7.2**).

As a result of these findings, standard-dose amoxicillin (40-60 mg/kg/d) could be considered for older patients and patients at low risk for infection with PNSP, but high-dose amoxicillin is recommended for those at greater risk for PNSP.[8-10,12] We believe that

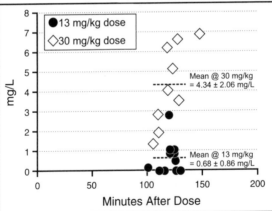

FIGURE 7.2 — Amoxicillin Concentrations in Middle Ear Fluid* After Oral Doses of 13 or 30 mg/kg Amoxicillin Suspension for Acute Otitis Media[†]

- 13 mg/kg dose
- ◇ 30 mg/kg dose

Mean @ 30 mg/kg = 4.34 ± 2.06 mg/L

Mean @ 13 mg/kg = 0.68 ± 0.86 mg/L

* Obtained by tympanocentesis and subjected to assays for amoxicillin concentrations.
† The National Committee on Clinical Laboratory Standards "susceptibility break point" of *Streptococcus pneumoniae* for amoxicillin is 2 µg/mL.

Harrison CJ, Welch DF. *Pediatr Infect Dis J.* 1998;17:657-658.

practitioners should consider avoiding doses <30 mg/kg/dose of amoxicillin to ensure reasonable MEE concentrations of drug in all patients. However, no clinical trial data have shown superior effectiveness of high-dose over standard-dose amoxicillin.

■ Rationale for 10-Day Course

A full 10-day course of amoxicillin is recommended for children who are younger than 2 or 3 years or who are at higher risk for PNSP. A 5- to 7-day course of amoxicillin should be adequate for older children at low risk for PNSP.[13] In children who are >2 years of age, standard-dose amoxicillin may be reasonable.

Why are 10 days of treatment preferred for younger or otitis-prone patients? Effective antibiotics usually sterilize MEE or suppress bacterial growth by 4 to 6 days,[14,15] so 4 to 6 days would seem adequate. Even younger and otitis-prone patients have sterile MEE at 4 to 6 days of therapy. But the data from well-conducted clinical studies of children <2 years of age or otitis-prone children show that 10-day therapy with β-lactams is often superior to 5-day therapy.[16] Another advantage of 10-day therapy occurs because children with poor eustachian tube function (<2 years of age or otitis-prone) tend to become reinfected in the 4 to 6 days after antibiotics have initially sterilized the MEE. Thus the additional 4 to 6 days of antibiotics theoretically may prevent reinfection with the same pathogen (still in the nasopharynx) or a new pathogen, until inflammation decreases sufficiently to allow mechanical factors to protect the middle ear space better. Alternatively, one could postulate that slower-acting drugs or more resistant pathogens require longer than 6 days for resolution of the AOM.

Some clinicians consider a child to be allergic to a drug if he or she has a rash during therapy with the drug. However, this type of "drug rash" frequently is virally induced and may not indicate hypersensitivity. Signs most likely to support true drug allergy include:

- Urticaria
- Pruritic rash
- Arthralgia
- Any signs of anaphylaxis.

Erythema multiforme (major or minor) and angioedema are other nonallergic hypersensitivity reactions that are a reasonable cause to avoid a particular antibiotic in the future.

For the child with AOM who is truly allergic to penicillins (<5% of children), the following are first-choice antibiotics: (**Figure 7.3**)[17]:

- A macrolide (azithromycin)
- A cephalosporin (cefdinir or cefpodoxime) (cefprozil would no longer be a reasonable choice for PCV-7 children who have a preponderance of *H influenzae*).
- Trimethoprim/sulfamethoxazole (TMP/SMX) is least preferred by most clinicians and lacks sufficient *H influenzae* coverage for PCV-7–vaccinated children.[18]

For the child who is severely allergic to penicillin (anaphylaxis or angioedema) and to all β-lactam drugs (cephalosporins as well as penicillins), choices include a macrolide antibiotic, such as azithromycin (preferred) or clarithromycin. TMP/SMX and erythromycin-sulfisoxazole are no longer reasonable choices for children who have received PCV-7 due to lack of coverage of *H influenzae*.[7,12,18]

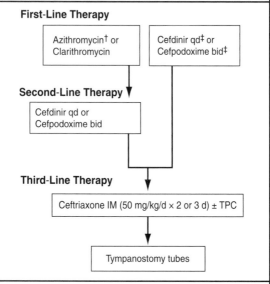

FIGURE 7.3 — Antibiotic Choices for Acute Otitis Media in the Nonseverely Penicillin-Allergic Child in the 2000s*

First-Line Therapy

Azithromycin† or Clarithromycin

Cefdinir qd‡ or Cefpodoxime bid‡

Second-Line Therapy

Cefdinir qd or Cefpodoxime bid

Third-Line Therapy

Ceftriaxone IM (50 mg/kg/d × 2 or 3 d) ± TPC

Tympanostomy tubes

Abbreviations: IM, intramuscularly; TPC, tympanocentesis with culture and susceptibility testing.

* Recommendations are for children 3 to 36 months old with acute otitis media (AOM).
† As azithromycin's coverage of *H influenzae* is limited (~50%); also AOM with concomitant pneumonia suggestive of atypical pathogens. Use of one of the newly approved regimens (10 mg/kg/day × 3 days or 30 mg/kg as one dose) is preferred. Lower success rates might be expected for macrolide/azalide therapy for AOM in the era of increasing prevalence of *H influenzae* as the cause of AOM (post pneumococcal conjugate vaccine [PCV-7]–use).
‡ Also AOM with concomitant conjunctivitis.

Because of the limited number of efficacious antibiotics available, these children will more likely eventually require pressure-equalizing (PE) tube insertion.

First-Line Therapy for the Child With Decreased Immune System Function

An antibiotic with an extended spectrum of activity is more appropriate than narrow-spectrum amoxicillin for children with decreased immune system function and/or those who have received chronic antibiotics prophylaxis, including treatments for diseases such as[19]:

- Sickle cell disease
- Immunodeficiency, primary or acquired (AIDS)
- Chemotherapy or chronic corticosteroid therapy
- Recurrent urinary tract infection
- Rheumatic fever.

If amoxicillin is chosen, these children should be treated with higher doses. But a second-line agent is preferred if they are already receiving amoxicillin prophylaxis.

■ For the Child With Suspected Pneumococcal Bacteremia Plus AOM

Children with suspected bacteremia who are not toxic and appear mildly to minimally ill may be treated with high-dose amoxicillin. For those who are more ill but not toxic, parenteral ceftriaxone is the preferred agent. A blood culture should be obtained before prescribing either antibiotic. Occult pneumococcal bacteremia has become much less common secondary to the adequate supply and routine use of PCV-7.[20,21] In a large HMO in northern California, no cases of vaccine serotype disease were seen in children <1 year of age despite a lack of the full series of PCV-7 (less than the 3 or 4 age-appropriate doses). The rate of nonvaccine serotypes causing invasive disease did not increase correspondingly.[20] Regardless, phone contact and follow-up must be assured and the child's condition must be assessed within 24 hours.

Likewise, in a postmarketing study of PCV-7 efficacy against invasive pneumococcal disease, marked reductions were noted in all age groups. Similar reductions were seen in children <5 years of age, but it was a marked reduction for all ages. No serotype substitution was noted in the first 2 years after the patients were immunized.[20] Unlike *H influenzae* type B (HIB) vaccine and HIB disease, pneumococcal invasive disease will not be vanquished by PCV-7, and it must still be a consideration in mild to moderately ill febrile children, just as it is for the toxic child.

REFERENCES

1. Casey JR, Pichichero ME. Changes in frequency and pathogens causing acute otitis media in 1995-2003. *Pediatr Infect Dis J.* 2004;23:824-828.

2. Block SL, Hedrick J, Harrison CJ, et al. Community-wide vaccination with the heptavalent pneumococcal conjugate significantly alters the microbiology of acute otitis media. *Pediatr Infect Dis J.* 2004;23:829-833.

3. American Academy of Pediatrics Subcommittee on Management of Acute Otitis Media. Diagnosis and management of acute otitis media. *Pediatrics.* 2004;113:1451-1465.

4. Garbutt J, St Geme JW 3rd, May A, Storch GA, Shackelford PG. Developing community-specific recommendations for first-line treatment of acute otitis media: is high-dose amoxicillin necessary? *Pediatrics.* 2004;114:342-347.

5. Rodriguez WJ, Schwartz RH. *Streptococcus pneumoniae* causes otitis media with higher fever and more redness of tympanic membranes than *Haemophilus influenzae* or *Moraxella catarrhalis. Pediatr Infect Dis J.* 1999;18:942-944.

6. Sclar DA, Tartaglione TA, Fine MJ. Overview of issues related to medical compliance with implications for the outpatient management of infectious diseases. *Infect Agents Dis.* 1994;3:266-273.

7. Dowell SF, Butler JC, Giebink GS, et al. Acute otitis media: management and surveillance in an era of pneumococcal resistance-a report from the Drug-resistant Streptococcus pneumoniae Therapeutic Working Group. *Pediatr Infect Dis J.* 1999;18:1-9.

8. Harrison CJ, Welch DF. Middle ear effusion amoxicillin concentrations in acute otitis media. *Pediatr Infect Dis J.* 1998;17:657-658.

9. Lister PD, Pong A, Chartrand SA, Sanders CC. Rationale behind high-dose amoxicillin therapy for acute otitis media due to penicillin-nonsusceptible pneumococci: support from in vitro pharmacodynamic studies. *Antimicrob Agents Chemother.* 1997;41:1926-1932.

10. Canafax DM, Yuan Z, Chonmaitree T, Deka K, Russlie HQ, Giebink GS. Amoxicillin middle ear fluid penetration and pharmacokinetics in children with acute otitis media. *Pediatr Infect Dis J.* 1998;17:149-156.

11. Seikel K, Shelton S, McCracken GH. Middle ear fluid concentrations of amoxicillin after large dosages in children with acute otitis media. *Pediatr Infect Dis J.* 1997;16:710-711.

12. Klein JO. Review of consensus reports on management of acute otitis media. *Pediatr Infect Dis J.* 1999;18:1152-1155.

13. Kozyrskyj AL, Hildes-Ripstein GE, Longstaffe SE, et al. Treatment of acute otitis media with a shortened course of antibiotics: a meta-analysis. *JAMA.* 1998;279:1736-1742.

14. Dagan R, Johnson CE, McLinn S, et al. Bacteriologic and clinical efficacy of amoxicillin/clavulanate vs azithromycin in acute otitis media. *Pediatr Infect Dis J.* 2000;19:95-104.

15. Dagan R, Leibovitz E, Fliss DM, et al. Bacteriologic efficacies of oral azithromycin and oral cefaclor in treatment of acute otitis media in infants and young children. *Antimicrob Agents Chemother.* 2000;44:43-50.

16. Hoberman A, Paradise JL, Cohen R. Duration of therapy for acute otitis media. *Pediatr Infect Dis J.* 2000;19:471-473.

17. Pichichero ME. A review of evidence supporting the American Academy of Pediatrics recommendation for prescribing cephalosporin antibiotics for penicillin-allergic patients. *Pediatrics.* 2005;115:1048-1057.

18. Block SL. Management of acute otitis media in the 1990s. The decade of resistant pneumococcus. *Paediatr Drugs.* 1999;1:31-50.

19. Paradise JL. Managing otitis media: a time for change. *Pediatrics.* 1995;96:712-715.

20. Black S, Shinefield H, Baxter R, et al. Postlicensure surveillance for pneumococcal invasive disease after use of heptavalent pneumococcal conjugate vaccine in Northern California Kaiser Permanente. *Pediatr Infect Dis J.* 2004;23:485-489.

21. Whitney CG, Farley MM, Hadler J, et al, for the Active Bacterial Core Surveillance of the Emerging Infections Program Network. Decline in invasive pneumococcal disease after the introduction of protein-polysaccharide conjugate vaccine. *N Engl J Med.* 2003;348:1737-1746.

8

Second-Line and Third-Line Antibiotic Therapy

Second- or third-line therapy for acute otitis media (AOM) is indicated when AOM is:

- Persistent/refractory
- Recurrent (recent antibiotic therapy within 30 days).
- A culture-proven infection with a resistant pathogen.

Factors that may contribute to antibiotic failure are listed in **Table 8.1**.[1,2]

When a child develops AOM within a month of completing a prior antibiotic regimen for AOM, it might appear that the current AOM could have been a treatment failure. But recent data indicate that this is true for only 28% of patients in whom therapy has failed within the first 7 days.[3] However, the actual percentage of relapse vs the percentage of new pathogens varied for different intervals of time after cessation of therapy (**Table 8.2**). Therefore, at most, only half are true treatment failures whereas the remainder are failures of the host, ie, the dysfunctional eustachian tube with residual inflammation allowing reinfection with a new pathogen.

Options for Therapy

■ **American Academy of Pediatrics/ American Academy of Family Physicians (AAP/AAFP) Guideline**

The AAP/AAFP guideline recommends amoxicillin/ clavulanate 90 mg/6.4 mg/kg/day as the only antibac-

TABLE 8.1 — Possible Factors Contributing to Failure of Antibiotic Therapy for Acute Otitis Media

Microbiology/Pharmacology "Mismatch"
- Pathogen resistant to selected antibiotic
  - Inadequate spectrum of activity for pathogen (eg, trimethoprim/sulfamethoxazole (TMP/SMX) for *Streptococcus pyogenes*, cefixime for penicillin-nonsusceptible *S pneumoniae* [PNSP])
  - Uncommon pathogen (eg, *Chlamydia pneumoniae*)
  - Coinfection with nonsusceptible pathogen (eg, β-lactamase–producing organisms)
- Concomitant viral infection not affected by antibiotics
- Inadequate middle ear effusion concentration of antibiotic drug (too low dosage or host factors)

Host Factors
- Impaired host defenses (decreased immune system function)
- Adenoidal or nasopharyngeal reservoir of organism
- Poor eustachian tube function (increased anatomic and physiologic risk factors)
- Poor compliance
- Reduced antibiotic absorption (may be due to gastroenteritis or antibiotic-induced hypermotility)
- Enhanced metabolism or excretion of active form of antibiotic

Environmental Factors
- Day care attendance (exposure to viral or bacterial reinfection)
- Smoking in the household

Data from: Block SL. *Paediatr Drugs*. 1999;1:31-50; Blumer JL. *Pediatr Infect Dis J*. 1999;18:1130-1140.

terial agent to be used for patients in whom initial management with an antibacterial agent failed.[4]

■ **Our Perspective**

To limit the single antibiotic choice for second-line therapy to amoxicillin/clavulanate, which has

TABLE 8.2 — Recurrent Acute Otitis Media:

TABLE 8.2 — Recurrent Acute Otitis Media: Percentage of Treatment Failure vs New Infection With New Pathogen		
Time Post-Therapy (days)	**Relapse (Failure) (%)**	**New Pathogen (%)**
0-7	46	54
8-14	32	68
15-21	24	76
22-28	11	89
Leibovitz E, et al. *Pediatr Infect Dis J.* 2003;22:209-216.		

some significant rates of adverse effects and palatability problems, is too restrictive. Other choices appear to be needed. We believe two broad-spectrum third-generation oral cephalosporins, cefdinir and cefpodoxime, are also reasonable second-line choices for amoxicillin failures given the recent increase in β-lactamase–producing *Haemophilus influenzae* and the decrease in penicillin-nonsusceptible *Streptococcus pneumoniae* (PNSP). We believe that our algorithm shown in **Figure 6.4** provides the practitioner with reasonable antibiotic choices.

These two third-generation cephalosporins have excellent activity against gram-negative and β-lactamase–producing organisms and reasonable coverage for activity against intermediately resistant PNSP. This is especially important in light of the microbiologic shift to gram-negative organisms as the predominant pathogens of AOM in young children.[5,6] These two antibiotics provide some compliance and tolerability advantages along with particularly high activity against gram-negative otopathogens.

Cefdinir also has recently proved to have superior taste, dosing (once daily), and tolerability. In a recent clinical trial, short-course cefdinir (5 days) also showed efficacy comparable to a full 10 days of low-dose amoxicillin/clavulanate.[7] In the overall study population, among children vaccinated with PCV-7, cefdinir was superior in efficacy compared with amoxicillin/clavulanate for those 6 months to 6 years (92% vs 82%, 95% CI [1.1, 18.4], $P = 0.024$) and for those 6 months the 24 months (92% vs 77%, 95% CI [3.5, 26.2], $P = 0.02$). Because the wide 95% CI occurred due to the smaller sample size for those 6 to 24 months, this precludes any definitive recommendations for this age group specifically.

We have not emphasized the use of cefuroxime (and possibly cefpodoxime) as second-line agents. We are concerned that cefuroxime (and cefpodoxime) has major taste problems. Neither cefpodoxime nor cefuroxime has undergone comparative clinical trials in the United States since the high prevalence of PNSP in AOM or the routine institution of pneumococcal conjugate vaccine (PCV)–7 in the childhood vaccination series with its subsequent microbiologic shift toward *H influenzae*.

As shown in the algorithm for treatment of AOM (**Figure 6.4**), recommendations for second- and third-line therapy of AOM in children without penicillin allergy are as follows:

- High-dose amoxicillin/clavulanate at 90 mg/kg amoxicillin with 6.4 mg/kg clavulanate per day (Augmentin ES)
- Cefdinir once a day (14 mg/kg/day)
- Cefpodoxime twice a day (10 mg/kg/day)
- If a young child has been fully vaccinated with PCV-7, the child has modest "mucosal" protection against the seven most common strains of *S pneumoniae*, particularly the most common PNSP strains (6B, 9V, 14, 19F, and 23F). Although we have significant reservations, some believe that cefixime could be considered for second-line therapy in such a child without high

fever or otalgia. Note that at least 30% of AOM pathogens remaining in refractory AOM are *S pneumoniae*. Cefixime lacks activity against PNSP.

Pneumococcal Conjugate Vaccine and Prevention of AOM

The Food and Drug Administration (FDA) has approved PCV-7, known as Prevnar, for prevention of pneumococcal invasive disease and AOM. This vaccine contains the nontoxic diphtheria-toxin analogue CRM197 conjugated to capsular polysaccharides from seven serotypes, five of which caused the majority of invasive disease and also AOM in the era before routine PCV-7 use. It was originally approved in February 2000 for prevention of invasive pneumococcal disease. Since then, it has been recommended for universal immunization of children <2 years old and for other high-risk unvaccinated patients up to 5 years old. Despite its approval for AOM prevention, it has not prevented AOM—a mucosal disease—with near the efficiency as it does invasive disease. This is in part because higher serum antibody levels may be required to prevent mucosal disease, and only a portion of AOM is due to pneumococcus, so a pneumococcal vaccine cannot be expected to prevent all AOM. For example, if one assumes that in unimmunized children *S pneumoniae* causes ~35% of all AOM and PCV-7 contains ~70% of the serotypes that cause AOM, then the maximum reduction in total episodes of AOM that we can expect (even if the vaccine is 100% effective in protecting against each of the PCV-7 strains) would be $70\% \times 35\% = 24\%$.

Vaccines are not expected to be 100% effective against infections at the mucosal surface where the antibodies induced by intramuscular (as opposed to mucosally applied) vaccines are likely to be 10-fold

161

less than antibody concentrations in serum/blood. So one would predict a more potent reliable protection against invasive (blood-borne bacteremia/sepsis or meningitis) than mucosal (AOM or sinusitis) infections. The data on PCV-7 in clinical trials investigating invasive disease and AOM prevention confirm this. Still, the preventive effects have caused a modest but significant reduction in recalcitrant AOM, AOM due to PNSP, and tympanostomy tube placement for recurrent AOM.

■ Clinical Studies
Invasive Disease

The data from clinical trials that led to FDA approval for prevention of invasive disease were dramatic and impressive. In the landmark Kaiser-Permanente double-blind study, there was ~95% reduction in invasive disease due to PCV-7 strains among those of the 37,868 enrolled children given PCV-7 at 2, 4, 6, and 12 to 15 months of age.[8] In a later evaluation in a northern California HMO, over 150,000 children had received one or more doses of PCV-7 but only 24% of those younger than 2 years of age received all four doses due to vaccine shortages. During the last year of observation, no cases of vaccine serotype disease were seen in children <1 year old compared with a prior incidence of 16 to 34 cases annually. No concomitant increase in nonvaccine serotype pneumococcal invasive disease was observed.[9]

AOM Due to Pneumococcus

The initial Kaiser-Permanente study[8] revealed the following reductions in AOM: 7% for AOM overall, 64.7% for AOM due to serotypes found in the PCV-7, but only in children with spontaneous otorrhea, 22.8% for recurrent AOM, and 20.1% in pressure-equalizing (PE) tube placement. The caveat was that the 64.7%

reduction was based on a subset of only 23 children with culture-proven pneumococcal AOM presenting as spontaneously perforated AOM.

In a Finnish randomized, double-blind efficacy trial of 1,662 infants with the same vaccine given at 2, 4, 6, and 12 months of age,[10] reductions were 6% (95%, confidence interval [CI] = –4%–16%) for AOM overall in 6- to 24-month-old subjects. The negative value for the lower CI number indicates that the actual outcome could have been anywhere from a 4% increase to a 16% reduction in AOM. More encouraging was the 34% (95% CI 21%–45%) decrease in culture-confirmed AOM due to any pneumococcus, and 57% (95 CI 44%–67%) reduction due to PCV-7 serotypes. Further, AOM due to PCV-7 cross-reacting pneumococci also decreased 51%.

8

Overall AOM Reduction

Highly experienced investigators from rural Kentucky studied two cohorts of an entire clinic population of children from birth to 36 months, reporting on rates of AOM and overall antibiotic days. Nearly 94% of all children in the practice in the cohort born after June 2000 had been vaccinated with three or four doses of PCV-7; >90% of the population was white and the majority of the children attended day care. They observed a 19% overall reduction in AOM for the first 3 years of life and a 28% reduction in overall antibiotic days. They attributed most of the higher reduction in rates of AOM to the "herd immunity" effects of having the entire population of young cohorts vaccinated.[11,12]

Similarly, two populations of young children (Tennessee Medicaid program consisting of mostly ethnic minority and a mostly white population in suburban Rochester, NY) were studied for rates of AOM before and after the introduction of PCV-7.[13] The rates of reduction for overall AOM were 6% and 20%, respectively. The reduction in the suburban, mostly white population almost mirrored the rural Kentucky findings, suggesting that a much large impact of PCV-7 seems to occur in children who are more otitis prone[11] and in day care (see Chapter 2, *Epidemiology*).

Serotype Substitution

About 90 other serotypes of pneumococcus are known. Some questions exist as to whether PCV-7 prevention of AOM due to these seven serotypes will open the door for other serotypes to begin causing AOM (known as serotype substitution). In a Finnish study, AOM due to non–PCV-7 strains increased 33%, so some serotype substitution might occur in everyday practice.[10] This substitution was confirmed in Pittsburgh, with the proportion of nonvaccine serotypes rising from 21% to 47% of isolates.[14]

At first glance, serotype substitution may appear to blunt the benefit of PCV-7. But this phenomenon may more likely be a proportional, and not an absolute, increase in non–PCV-7 strains. Non–PCV-7 pathogens are also much less likely to be PNSP (**Figure 8.1**). Therefore the "new" AOM serotypes are still much more likely to be penicillin susceptible and more easily eradicated with standard oral drugs. These non–PCV-7 serotypes also appear less likely to be invasive. The occasional bacteremia or meningitis sequelae of pneumococcal AOM may also be reduced. More recently, overall proportions of *S pneumoniae* isolates and vaccine serotypes in AOM were significantly reduced by community-wide use of PCV-7 vaccine in Kentucky.[12] Also, proportions of gram-negative AOM pathogens (predominantly nontypeable *H influenzae*) became 2-fold more frequent than *S pneumoniae* after PCV-7 vaccination.[5]

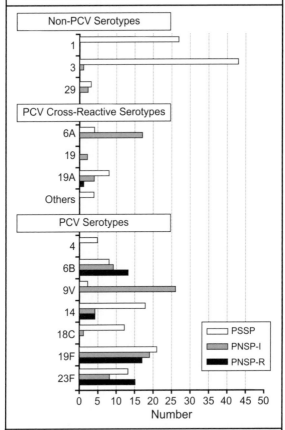

FIGURE 8.1 — Serotype Distribution in Relation to Penicillin Susceptibility of Pneumococcal Isolates From Acute Otitis Media: 1992-1998

Abbreviations: non-PCV, nonvaccine serotypes; PCV, pneumococcal conjugate vaccine; PNSP, penicillin-nonsusceptible *Streptococcus pneumoniae*; PNSP-I, intermediate PNSP (penicillin minimum inhibitory concentration [MIC] 0.2–1.0 µg/mL); PNSP-R, resistant PNSP (penicillin MIC ≥2.0 µg/mL); PSSP, penicillin-susceptible *S pneumoniae*.

Adapted from: Block SL, et al. *Pediatr Infect Dis J*. 2002; 21:859-865.

Nasopharynx Colonization After PCV-7

Most pneumococcal AOM cases result from pneumococci that have recently colonized the nasopharynx (NP) of young children. One relatively noninvasive way to monitor for serotype substitution is through NP surveillance of young immunized children to see whether colonization with PCV-7 strains decrease and non–PCV-7 strains increase over time. Several studies have already looked into this and others are under way. In Israel where PCV-7 is not routinely available, investigators studied NP colonization in a small subpopulation of 264 children given a 9-valent PCV (PCV-9). This nonvalent PCV showed the highest reduction of carriage in 12- to 24-month old children and no reduction in children 4 to 6 years of age.[15] However, serotype 19F was not reduced at any age. Non–PCV-9 strains increased only 10% compared with controls.

One of the authors has also seen a decrease in NP colonization with PCV-7 strains in 2002-2003 from 23% to 6% and an accompanying 10% increase in non–PCV-7 strains (Harrison CJ, Jones VF. In press; Harrison CJ, et al. SPR abstract, 2002). Another concern in the era of emerging methicillin-resistant *Staphylococcus aureus* (MRSA) is the increased MRSA NP colonization in PCV-7–immunized children in whom PCV-7 serotypes were absent. This may be a negative PCV-7 effect. Non–PCV-7 strains appear to cohabit with MRSA, whereas the presence of MRSA was more likely to be reduced in the NP if PCV-7 strains were the predominant NP colonizer.[16]

To cover for new serotypes causing AOM or other diseases, additional important serotypes are being added to the current vaccine. The most likely PCV to be available and which is currently undergoing testing in the United States will likely contain 13 serotypes. Most importantly, it will include serotypes 6A and 19A, which still do not appear to be adequately covered in mucosal disease with PCV-7 and which are commonly PNSP.[5]

■ Potential Large-Scale Impact of Vaccine

AOM is one of the most common bacterial infections in children, affecting >60% of all US children during the first year of life and 94% by the age of 3 years. It leads to about 25 million physician office visits and costs the US health care system and society up to $5 billion every year. A 7% reduction in AOM would reduce annual AOM expenditures by $350 million. Similarly, reduced placement of PE tubes yields an additional $500 million savings. In the NY data from Poehling and associates in the subset of children from Rochester who were mostly white children,[13] the rate of reduction of episodes of AOM was nearly 20%, similar to a report from rural Kentucky in predominantly white children as well.[12] These numbers differ somewhat from the northern California data, which showed an estimated 8.9% reduction in the first 2 years of life.

Practitioners must realize that the third dose in the first 6 months of life seems to confer significantly better protection against AOM (mucosal disease) for the first 12 months of life. Also PCV-7 was most effective during 15 to 18 months of age shortly after the booster dose, when PCV-7 children had 12.2% fewer AOM visits than control children.[17] Tympanostomy tube placement was also reduced by 24% in the first 3.5 years of life (**Table 8.3**).[3] A recent study showed that only two priming doses at 2 and 4 months of age may suffice for protection against invasive disease. Use of such a schedule seems likely to reduce costs, a noble goal in the days of expanding health care costs. We are concerned that it may lead to more AOM due to PCV-7 in the 8- to 12-month age group. Intervals of >7 months between the last priming dose and the

TABLE 8.3 — Variation in the Effect of PCV on Otitis Visits by Race*

Subgroup	Otitis Visits/Year[†] (PCV/Control)	PCV Effect (% Reduction in Otitis Visits)	95% CI (Lower, Upper)
Asian	1.28/1.40	8.7	1.7, 15.0
Black	1.48/1.59	7.2	-2.3, 15.9
Hispanic	1.82/1.97	7.7	2.4, 12.7
Other, missing	1.64/1.75	5.8	-2.3, 13.2
White	2.11/2.29	8.0	4.7, 11.2

Abbreviation: CI, confidence interval; PCV, pneumococcal conjugate vaccine.

* $P = 0.986$; P value indicates the significant of variation in the PCV effect
† Visit rates are adjusted for age and season

Fireman B, et al. *Pediatr Infect Dis J.* 2003;22:10-16.

booster dose at 12 to 15 months of age has been shown to allow return of NP colonization with PCV-7 types.[18]

Selection Rationale of Second-Line Therapies for AOM

Previous data during the PNSP era (1990s) from children in whom amoxicillin has failed to clear AOM showed *S pneumoniae* to be the most common pathogen[11]:

- 26% penicillin-susceptible *S pneumoniae* (PSSP)
- 18% intermediate-level PNSP (PNSP-I)
- 13% high-level PNSP (PNSP-R).

However, with the routine universal use of PCV-7 in young children, the primary pathogens causing refractory AOM in children 6 to 24 months old have been gram-negative organisms, primarily *H influenzae.* (Note that these pathogens are nontypeable *H influenzae,* which are not a component of the HIB [type B] vaccine routinely administered to children.) Therefore only a small portion of pathogens recovered from refractory AOM are currently PNSP, with <6% being high-level PNSP.[5,6,19]

Many amoxicillin failures are likely due to host factors, eg, noncompliance, poor drug absorption, or failure of absorbed antibiotic to penetrate middle ear effusion (MEE), as has been shown in up to 20% of children in three prior reports[20-22] This skew toward *H influenzae* also likely reflects the high *in vivo* potency of amoxicillin with or without clavulanate against pneumococcus.

8

Determining Relative Potential for Success of Second-Line Therapies

Three currently FDA-approved oral antibiotics for children show the broadest level of *in vitro* activity against the major pathogens of AOM, including PNSP. They are:

- Amoxicillin/clavulanate
- Cefdinir
- Cefpodoxime.

However, unlike cefdinir and amoxicillin/clavulanate, there are no efficacy data for cefpodoxime against PNSP in a tympanocentesis trial.

In the pre-PNSP era (1991-1992), from a multicenter clinical tympanocentesis trial of children 6 months old to 12 years old with AOM undergoing a single tympanocentesis, Block and colleagues reported that 10 days of once-daily cefdinir was as clinically effective as traditional-dose amoxicillin/clavulanate (40/10) tid for 10 days.[23,24] This study also showed a higher cure rate for 10 days of either the once-daily (14 mg/kg qd) vs the bid (7 mg/kg bid) dosing of cefdinir in children <2 years old (78% vs 66.7%) (*P* <0.05). A short course (5 days) of cefdinir bid was as effective as 10 days cefprozil bid in a nontympanocentesis study. Neither of these studies involved children with refractory AOM.

A recent international multicenter double-tap study that was unblinded, nonrandomized, and noncomparative, suggested that the high-dose formulation of amoxicillin/clavulanate (90 mg/6.4 mg/kg/day) administered bid was highly effective against PNSP-R. Pneumococcus was confirmed as eradicated (sterile middle ear fluid) by day 4 to 6 in >90% of the intent-to-treat patients. In this study, higher doses of amoxicillin (90 mg/kg/day) divided bid eradicated

PNSP with minimum inhibitory concentrations (MICs) up to 4 mg/mL.

Thus far, no double-tap clinical trial data have examined the efficacy of low dose amoxicillin/clavulanate (40 mg:10 mg or 45 mg:6.4 mg/kg/day) or oral cephalosporins against PNSP-R.[25] There have been relatively few reports in the United States of efficacy rates achieved by various antibiotics in small groups of children with persistent/refractory AOM after amoxicillin therapy. The results in these unblinded and nonrandomized studies showed that amoxicillin/clavulanate, cefprozil, and cefdinir had similar cure rates of 60% to 70% for AOM caused by PNSP.[26] However, like the double-tap data from Israel, the small number of PNSP strains and nonrandomized, nonblinded design of these studies provide a marginal basis for refractory AOM recommendations. Furthermore, cefprozil has inadequate *in vitro* coverage of activity against β-lactamase–producing *H influenzae* and *Moraxella catarrhalis*, suggesting high rates of failures would be likely among children vaccinated with PCV-7 who have predominantly gram-negative organisms (**Table 8.4**).

As for actual clinical *in vivo* data, the only clinical trial comparing high-dose amoxicillin/clavulanate with low-dose amoxicillin/clavulanate showed no difference in overall efficacy between the two formulations.[27] Only *in vitro* data suggest that high-dose amoxicillin/clavulanate should be superior to low-dose amoxicillin/clavulanate (see *Time Above MIC Data* section below).

Well-designed clinical studies with sufficient power to detect real differences in efficacy of second-line agents for antibiotic failures are lacking. Various pharmacologic markers have been used to try to predict which antibiotics will have the best activity against an AOM pathogen that has failed to respond to first-line therapy.

8

TABLE 8.4 — Likelihood of Various Antibiotics to Reach Effective MIC:MEE Ratios in MEE for Drug-Resistant and Drug-Susceptible Pathogens

| Antibiotic (dose, mg/kg) | Mean Peak MEE (mg/L) | MEE:MIC (Relative in vitro Activity) | | | | |
		PNSP-R ≥2.0 µg/mL	PNSP-I 0.1-1.0 µg/L	Haemophilus influenzae β-Lactamase(+)	Haemophilus influenzae β-Lactamase(−)	Moraxella catarrhalis (+)
Penicillins						
Amoxicillin (standard dose 60 mg/kg/d)	4.34	+	+++	—	+++	+
Amox/clav 7:1 (45 mg/kg/d)	5.6	+	+++	++++	++++	++++
Amoxicillin (high dose 80-100 mg/kg/d)	6.3	+++	++++	—	++++	+
Amox/clav (high dose 90 mg/kg/d)	6.3	+++	++++	++++	++++	++++
Cephalosporins						
Second-Generation						
Cefaclor	0.47-3.8	—	—	—	++	+++

Cefprozil	2.0	+	++	+	++++	++
Cefuroxime	1.2	+	++	+++	+++	+++
Third-Generation						
Cefdinir	0.71	+	++/+++	++++	++++	++++
Cefixime	0.35–2.86	–	–	++++	++++	++++
Cefpodoxime	0.49–0.87	+	++	+++	++++	++++
Ceftibuten	4.0	–	–	++++	++++	++
Ceftriaxone (×1)*	35	+	+++	++++	++++	++++
Ceftriaxone (×3)*	35	+++	++++	++++	++++	++++
Macrolides						
Azithromycin (10 mg/kg)	1.05–8.6[†]	+[‡]	++	++	++	++++
Azithromycin (30 mg/kg)	∞	∞	∞	∞	∞	∞
Clarithromycin	7.4 (11.2‖)[†]	+[‡]	++	+	+	++++

Continued

Antibiotic (dose, mg/kg)	Mean Peak MEE (mg/L)	MEE:MIC (Relative in vitro Activity)				
		PNSP-R ≥2.0 µg/mL	PNSP-I 0.1-1.0 µg/L	Haemophilus influenzae		Moraxella catarrhalis (+)
				β-Lactamase(+)	β-Lactamase(-)	
Other						
Clindamycin	3.6†	+++	++++	—	—	—
Erythromycin/ sulfisoxazole	0.5	++‡	++	+	+	+++
TMP/SMX (19:1)	1.39-2.0	—	—	+++	+++	+++

Abbreviations: Amox/clav, amoxicillin/clavulanate; IM, intramuscular; MEE, middle ear effusion; MIC, minimum inhibitory concentration; PNSP-I, intermediate-level penicillin-nonsusceptible *Streptococcus pneumoniae*; PNSP-R, resistant penicillin-nonsusceptible *S pneumoniae*; TMP/SMX, trimethoprim/sulfamethoxazole.

Key: —, none; +, <30% of organisms; ++, 30%-60% of organisms; +++, 60%-90% of organisms; +++, >90% of organisms.

* One dose IM is FDA approved for AOM therapy; however, the regimen of three doses is not.

† Concentration in extracellular MEE fluid is <10% of total. This may affect efficacy since replicating bacteria are only in extracellular MEE fluid.

‡ Lower values (+) were compared with 1992-1995 values, which were slightly higher (++).

§ There are no pharmacokinetic data on azithromycin 30 mg/kg as of the end of 2002. Therefore, predictions of increased efficacy compared with 10 mg/kg dosing cannot be made at present.

‖ Includes 14-OH clarithromycin metabolite.

Adapted from Block SL. *Paediatr Drugs.* 1999;1:31-50.

Relative Prevalence of Treatment-Resistant AOM Pathogens

In the 1980s, *H influenzae* appeared to be the most frequent cause of refractory/recurrent AOM (46% to 62% of cases).[28,29] In contrast, in the 1990s, most cases of AOM that failed to respond to multiple courses of antibiotics were caused by PNSP (30% to 91% of cases of recurrent AOM worldwide).[30-32] The availability in the United States since March 2000 of PCV-7 for immunization of children younger than 2 years has changed this trend. *H influenzae* has again become the most frequent cause of first-line therapy failure. PCV-7 is discussed more fully earlier in this chapter and in Chapter 11, *Prevention*. We shall discuss below the most frequent causes of amoxicillin failures as documented in the literature.

■ **Pathogen Target for Antibiotic Failures in Young Children With AOM**

The pathogen target for AOM failures in young children include:

- In the 1980s, β-lactamase-positive *H influenzae*[33]
- In the 1990s, PNSP and highly resistant PNSP[19]
- In the 2000s in PCV-7–vaccinated children, β-lactamase-positive *H influenzae*[5,6]
  - Note: <20% of pathogens in the 2000s are PNSP, with only 5% to 6% of those being highly resistant PNSP

■ **Amoxicillin Failures in AOM**

In the pre-PNSP era of the early 1990s, the primary pathogen isolated from an amoxicillin failure was *S pneumoniae*[34]; a later study during the PNSP era showed that it was still predominantly *S pneumoniae* with approximately half of strains as PNSP.[5] In the

2000s during the PCV-7 era, two studies from rural Kentucky and Rochester, NY, showed that the predominant pathogen of refractory/recurrent AOM is *H influenzae* with over half the strains producing β-lactamase.[5,6]

Let's assume that the practitioner has used high-dose amoxicillin as first-line therapy as recommended by the AAP/AAFP guideline. If high-dose amoxicillin has failed and the child has been vaccinated with PCV-7, we would assume that *H influenzae* would be the major target for antibiotic therapy. If the practitioner prescribed high-dose amoxicillin/clavulanate as second-line therapy, does this add any different *S pneumoniae* coverage or β-lactamase–negative *H influenzae* coverage? Not really.

If one selects a broad-spectrum third-generation cephalosporin at this juncture, these antibiotics target a different area (penicillin-binding protein [PBPs]) of *H influenzae,* thus providing unique added coverage above using an additional amino penicillin at this point.

AOM Clinical Trials in PCV-7–Vaccinated Children

Block and colleagues compared short-course (5-day) cefdinir bid with 10 days of low-dose amoxicillin/clavulanate (45 mg/6.4 mg/kg/day) bid in children with nonrefractory AOM.[7] These children had definitive findings of suppurative AOM. The trial was investigator blinded, multicenter, and nontympanocentesis, using clinical end points for efficacy rates. The mean age of children was 2.8 years (age range 6 months to 6 years) and two thirds of all children were vaccinated with PCV-7. At the end of therapy, the clinical success rate was 88% and 85% for cefdinir and amoxicillin/clavulanate, respectively.

In the subset of children who had received PCV-7, cefdinir was 10% more effective than amoxicillin/

clavulanate (92% vs 82%, $P = 0.024$, 95% CI = 1.1–18.4). In the subset of children age 6 to 24 months who had received PCV-7, cefdinir was 15% more effective than amoxicillin/clavulanate ($P = 0.019$, 95% CI = 3.5–26.2). These data suggest that among children who have received PCV-7, particularly in the younger cohort, cefdinir is highly efficacious, regardless of the antibiotic comparator.[5] The findings are most likely driven by the higher rates of *H influenzae* recovered from children who have received PCV-7 as suggested by two recent microbiologic surveillance studies of AOM.

The time-above-MIC data for all strains of *H influenzae* as calculated by Jacobs and Pelton[35,36] would corroborate these findings (cefdinir—81% [using cefpodoxime as a surrogate marker] and low-dose amoxicillin/clavulanate—42%) (**Table 8.5**).

8

Predicting Drug Efficacy Based on Pharmacokinetics and Pharmacodynamics

Because there are so few head-to-head well-designed AOM treatment studies, we need other tools to predict the relative efficacy of drugs as resistance changes and new drugs are released. Pharmacologic characteristics of antibiotics can be used as surrogate markers of efficacy combining MIC data with pharmacokinetic data (pharmacodynamics) and verifying predictions in an animal model:

- The first step is to evaluate a drug's pharmacokinetic properties (how the drug acts in the body), including:
  - Drug absorption (serum concentration at various times after dosing)
  - Drug distribution (concentration in MEE, determined by tympanocentesis)

TABLE 8.5 — Susceptibility for *Haemophilus influenzae**

Antibiotic	MEE Concentration	MIC 50	MIC 90	Time > MIC[†]
Amoxicillin/clavulanate (low/high dose)	2-4/4-6	1.0	2.0	41%/72%
Cefuroxime	0.6	0.5	1.0	33%
Cefprozil	2	4	16	21%
Cefdinir/Cefpodoxime	0.72	0.25	0.5	82%:?
Ceftriaxone	35-19 (2 day)	0.06	0.06	100%
Azithromycin	8.6	2	8	‡
TMP/SMX	1.4-2.0	0.12	4	0%-20%

Abbreviations: MEE, middle ear effusion; MIC, minimum inhibitory concentration; TMP/SMX, trimethoprim/sulfamethoxazole

* T>MIC of 40% = good penicillin antibiotic.

† Based on serum concentrations of specific antibiotics.

‡ Azithromycin's pharmacodynamic requirement is not Time >MIC but area under the curve (AUC)/MIC ratio of >30 for gram-positive pathogens and >125 for gram-negative pathogens. The AUC of protein-unbound plasma azithromycin is the datum used for these calculations.

Jacobs MR. *Clin Microbiol Infect.* 2001;7:589-596; Long SS, Pickering LK, Prober CG, eds. *Principles and Practice of Pediatric Infectious Diseases.* 2nd ed. Philadelphia, Pa: Churchill Livingstone; 2002.

- Drug metabolism (may be affected by food and other disease)
- Drug excretion (may affect or be affected by kidney or liver function)

- The second step is to define the drug's pharmacodynamic properties (how drug activity affects specific pathogens) using evaluations of time-kill assays and postantibiotic effects.

- The third step is *in vivo* investigation using animal models (eg, William Craig's mouse model) to confirm pharmacodynamic predictions. Pharmacodynamic efficacy depends on:
  - Mechanism of action (eg, inhibit protein synthesis/macrolide) or prevent cell wall synthesis (β-lactam)
  - Exceeding a concentration in MEE long enough or by a sufficient amount for the drug action to take place.

In addition, the formulation of a drug (eg, suspension versus tablet, oral vs intramuscular injection, one manufacturer vs another) also may produce different effects or modify properties. For example, palatability or dosing schedule can affect efficacy indirectly by decreasing or increasing patient compliance with therapy.

In Vivo Measures of Antibiotic Efficacy

In 1969, Howie and Ploussard reported on a "double-tap" technique (tympanocentesis before the start and again midway through antibiotic therapy) to measure directly how well antibiotics eliminated bacteria midtherapy from the middle ear.[37] However, tympanocentesis is uncomfortable for the child, relatively time-consuming, and expensive. In addition, subsequent research has shown that failure to sterilize the middle ear fluid on day 4 to 6 of therapy ("failure of bacteriologic cure") does not always predict clinical failure, but rates of clinical cure are less than when bacteriologic eradication does occur (25% to 60% vs >90% clinical cure).[37-40] Very few families in the United States will allow their child to undergo double-tap. Consequently, most data used to estimate antibiotic efficacy *in vivo* are obtained in "single-tap" studies in which a sample of MEE is obtained by tympanocentesis before dosing with antibiotic. However, double-tap studies are the best estimates of rapid elimination of the pathogen based mostly on the drug effect and the bacteriostatic vs bacteriocidal nature of the drug. Clinical response rates in nontap and single-tap studies take into account drug effects that may occur after day 6 of therapy. These include effects of slower-acting drugs, eg, bacteriostatic drugs, effects on high inoculum infections (it can take longer to eradicate 10^6 pathogens[6] in MEE than 10^3[3]), and the effects of spontaneous cures (nondrug effect).

Nontap AOM studies, however, do not provide information on the proportions of pathogens in the study patients or the number of drug-resistant pathogens. Therefore, applying the results to one's practice may be less reliable. Extreme care is needed to interpret success rates because these studies often exclude difficult-to-treat patients and include higher rates of older patients so that the outcomes are skewed toward higher success rates.

■ Pharmacokinetic Markers (Concentrations in Serum and Middle Ear Effusion)

One step in predicting whether an antibiotic will be effective in eradicating AOM pathogens is to determine what concentration the drug achieves in the MEE. **Table 8.6** shows the results of a meta-analysis of studies reporting on antibiotic concentrations in serum and MEE after single or multiple doses of antibiotics were used to treat AOM.[41]

Some antibiotic doses shown in **Table 8.6** were evaluated in more than one study, and in most cases, the results differ noticeably. The relationship between serum and MEE concentration of antibiotic also varied. Sources of variation include[42,43]:

- Timing of specimen collection after dosing
- Drug assay method
- Type, quality, and quantity of MEE (ie, concentrations of clarithromycin and azithromycin in purulent fluid from ears with AOM are three times higher than those in serous or mucoid effusions from ears with otitis media with effusion)
- Whether blood contaminated the MEE specimen (may overestimate the concentration of β-lactam antibiotics, trimethoprim/sulfamethoxazole, and some macrolides).

There are also variations by drug class due to differences in pharmacokinetics. The newer macrolides are absorbed rapidly and are distributed to intracellular sites more rapidly and completely than β-lactam drugs. Thus soon after dosing, macrolides will reach overall lower concentrations in serum and higher concentrations in MEE compared with β-lactam agents. However, concentrations of macrolides in the extracellular portion of MEE are <10% of the total MEE concentration. This may affect efficacy since replicating bacteria are almost exclusively in extracellular MEE fluid.

■ *In Vitro* **Pharmacodynamic Markers of Second-Line Therapy Agent Efficacy**

Antibiotics are not likely to be effective unless concentrations of active drug in MEE extracellular fluid exceed the MIC, minimum concentration of drug needed to inhibit growth for the AOM pathogen. For

TABLE 8.6 — Mean Peak Serum and Middle Ear Effusion Concentrations (µg/mL) of Some Antibiotics Used to Treat Acute Otitis Media

Antibiotic Class/Agent	Dose	Serum	MEE	MEE/Serum
Amoxicillin	13.3 mg/kg	11.2	2.8	0.25
	15 mg/kg	13.6	5.6	0.41
Cephalosporins				
Second-Generation				
Cefaclor	13.3 mg/kg	3.6	1.0	0.28
Cefprozil	15 mg/kg	8.5/16.8	0.5/3.8	0.06/0.23
Cefuroxime	15 mg/kg	5.5/12.1	2.0/2.0	0.36/0.17
Loracarbef	15 mg/kg/250 mg	5.1/5.4	0.2/1.2	0.22
	15 mg/kg	9.3	3.9	0.42
Third-Generation				
Cefdinir	14 mg/kg	4.11/3.60	0.72	0.15
Cefixime	8 mg/kg	2.5/4.2	1.3/1.5	0.52/0.36

Cefpodoxime	5 mg/kg		2.0	0.8	0.10
Ceftibuten	9 mg/kg		6.7/12.2	4.0/9.3	0.60/0.76
Macrolides					
Azithromycin	10-5-5-5-5 mg/kg	0.2		1.05/8.6/9.4*	43/47
Clarithromycin† 14-hydroxyclarithromycin†	7.5 mg/kg	3.42 1.77	8.3 2.9		2.0 1.66
Erythromycin ethylsuccinate	12.5 mg/kg	1.0	<0.2		<0.20
	15 mg/kg	1.20	0.5		0.42
Sulfisoxazole	37.5 mg/kg	106	20.9		0.20
Trimethoprim/sulfamethoxazole	4/20 mg/kg	2.0/44.6	1.4/8.2		0.70/0.18
	4/20 mg/kg	3.1/70.3	2.0/18.7		0.65/0.27

Abbreviation: MEE, middle ear effusion.

* At 24 and 48 hours.

† At 64 hours.

Data from meta-analysis by Craig WA, Andes D. *Pediatr Infect Dis J.* 1996;15:255-259; Guay DR. *Pediatr Infect Dis J.* 2000;19(suppl 12):S141-S146; Gan VN, et al. *Pediatr Infect Dis J.* 1997;16:39-43; *Physician's Desk Reference.* 59th ed. Monvale, NJ: Medical Economics Company; 2005. Entries formatted "x/y" indicate results from separate studies of the same drug dose.

8

this reason, the MEE:MIC ratio for a given antibiotic and pathogen is also a helpful surrogate for predicting drug efficacy. If peak MEE:MIC is >2, some efficacy is expected, and if it is >8, excellent efficacy is expected.

Exceeding the MIC in serum predicts success in bacteremia, but drugs distribute from serum to MEE in different ways. For β-lactams (penicillins and cephalosporins), less drug is found in MEE than in serum so that it can be helpful to calculate the ratio of penetration for different drugs. For example, 30% to 40% of amoxicillin serum concentrations are found in MEE and nearly all is in extracellular fluid. So if an amoxicillin serum level is 40 mg/mL, expect MEE to be 12 to 16 mg/mL. For azithromycin, however, serum concentrations are low and MEE concentrations tend to be 10 to 20 times higher, with nearly all found within inflammatory cells, away from replicating bacteria.

Using data obtained by tympanocentesis between 1992 and 1995 in a population of Kentucky children with AOM, Block calculated the relative *in vitro* activity, or MEE:MIC, for strains of *S pneumoniae*, *H influenzae*, and *M catarrhalis* (**Table 8.4**).[1] Data from 1998 to 2000 yielded similar outcome, but lower values were seen for macrolides and PNSP-R. Results of a similar analysis were formulated in a different format by Harrison (**Figure 8.2**).[42]

■ Surrogate Pharmacodynamic Markers of Drug Potential for Killing AOM Pathogens

Predicting *in vivo* drug activity against AOM pathogens would be easier if the concentration of drug in a serum sample could be used as a surrogate to predict the concentration of drug in MEE. Craig and Andes evaluated the relationship between drug concentration in serum and bacteriologic cure, using MEE:serum values from their meta-analysis.[41] The MEE and MIC data they used are predicated on tympanocentesis and culture of MEE on days 2 to 7 of antibiotic therapy. They predict that:

- Bacteriologic cure (>85% of bacteria in MEE eradicated) would be likely when serum drug concentrations exceeded the MIC for 40% to 50% of the dosing interval (40% for amoxicillin and 50% for cephalosporins). For example, if a drug was dosed every 12 hours and the MIC for the pathogen is 1.0 µg/mL, the penicillin drug would be expected to be effective if drug concentrations were >1.0 µg/mL for 4.8 hours (40% of 12-hour dosing interval). See **Figure 7.1** for a dosing curve for amoxicillin.
- Maximal killing (almost 100% sterilization of MEE) would be likely when MEE:MIC ratio was >10 at peak, which they calculated would result in serum:MIC being >1 for 60% to 70% of the dosing interval.

8

Time-Above-MIC Data

In the PCV-7 era, *H influenzae* accounts for over half the pathogens recovered from children with refractory/recurrent AOM, and high-level PNSP accounts for <6% of AOM pathogens in this group. We think that practitioners in the PCV-7 era need to become familiar with this concept, particularly for *H influenzae*.

Time-above-MIC data show that for *H influenzae*, cefprozil, cefuroxime, and TMP-SMX appear to provide unsatisfactory coverage. The three most active broad-spectrum antibiotics are high-dose amoxicillin/clavulanate, cefdinir, and cefpodoxime. Cefixime and ceftibuten provide minimal to no coverage for *S pneumoniae*, so they have not been included in this analysis.

Although Craig and Andes' calculations are valuable, using serum concentrations of drug to predict bacteriologic cure of AOM is dependent on serum and MEE concentration correlating reasonably well. Some drugs have low serum concentrations but concentrate

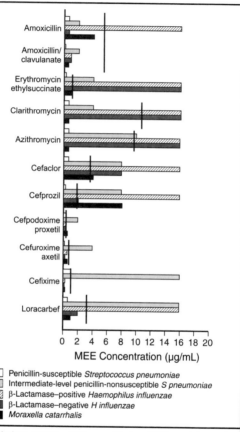

FIGURE 8.2 — MIC₉₀ Values of Antibiotics for Acute Otitis Media Pathogens Relative to Concentration of Drug in Middle Ear Effusion

Penicillin-susceptible *Streptococcus pneumoniae*
Intermediate-level penicillin-nonsusceptible *S pneumoniae*
β-Lactamase–positive *Haemophilus influenzae*
β-Lactamase–negative *H influenzae*
Moraxella catarrhalis

Abbreviations: MEE, middle ear effusion; MIC₉₀, minimum inhibitory concentration needed to inhibit growth of that pathogen by 90%.

Pathogens with MICs to the left of the vertical line for each drug are likely to be eradicated from the MEE by therapy with that drug. In contrast, pathogens with MICs to the right of the vertical line are likely to persist despite therapy with that drug.

Continued

NOTE: Cefdinir middle ear concentrations at 3 hours postdose of 14 mg/kg are 0.72 mg/L. The MIC_{90} for penicillin-susceptible *S pneumoniae* is 0.06 mg/L, for intermediate-level penicillin-nonsusceptible *S pneumoniae* is 1.0 mg/L, for β-lactamase–positive and negative *H influenzae* is 0.25 mg/L, and for *M catarrhalis*, 0.12 mg/L.

Modified from: Harrison CJ. *Pediatr Infect Dis J*. 1997;16:S12-S16.

well in MEE leukocytes (azithromycin) or penetrate MEE poorly (erythromycin ethyl succinate). Despite some limitations, pharmacodynamics give the best surrogate predictions of clinical success compared with any other method except large-scale clinical trials or double-tap studies.

■ Usefulness of Pharmacologic Markers in Selecting Second-Line Therapy for AOM

8

Success of an antibiotic in achieving bacteriologic cure of AOM (midtherapy) correlates reasonably well with success in achieving clinical cure (end of therapy). A drug's potential for achieving bacteriologic cure for persistent/refractory AOM is predicted by its *in vitro* activity against the particular drug-resistant pathogen.[23,24] Second-line therapies for AOM with >50% coverage for PNSP or β-lactamase–producing *H influenzae* or *M catarrhalis* are shown in **Table 8.4** and **Figure 8.2**.

Only the following second-line therapies provide good coverage for the two major resistant pathogens (PNSP and β-lactamase–producing *H influenzae*):

- Amoxicillin/clavulanate bid (high dose)
- Cefdinir qd
- Cefpodoxime bid (poor palatability)
- Ceftriaxone (two or three intramuscular [IM] doses).

In light of the time-above-MIC data for all strains of *H influenzae*, cefuroxime bid is not likely to provide

187

adequate coverage for children who have received PCV-7. In children who have been age-appropriately immunized with PCV-7, AOM failures may be more commonly caused by β-lactamase–producing *H influenzae*. Although cefixime does not have coverage for PNSP and only marginal coverage for PSSP, it has excellent coverage for β-lactamase–producing *H influenzae* and *M catarrhalis*.

Azithromycin Data in AOM

Azithromycin for second-line therapy in young children who have been fully immunized with PCV-7 may be suboptimal because of recent reports of waning coverage vs *H influenzae*. However, two recent clinical trials have shown that single-dose (30 mg/kg/dose) and high-dose azithromycin (20 mg/kg/day for 3 days) were equivalent to amoxicillin/clavulanate in a nontympanocentesis trial for new-onset AOM and tympanocentesis trial for persistent/recurrent AOM, respectively.[44,45]

When using azithromycin, the traditional 5-day course of 10 mg/kg, 5 mg/kg, 5 mg/kg, 5 mg/kg, and 5 mg/kg is no longer recommended. The recently approved 3-day dose (10 mg/kg qd) enhances the pharmacodynamic advantage for this drug by increasing the AUC/MIC for each 24-hour period. The one-dose regimen (30 mg/kg) certainly simplifies compliance issues but in clinical practice appears to precipitate a fair amount of gastrointestinal (GI) distress and vomiting, more so than reported in the clinical trial.[44] This probably occurred because no child in the clinical trial could have GI distress within a few days prior to entry in the study. A newer dose formulation of azithromycin (20 mg/kg/day for 3 days), which may be even better pharmacodynamically, showed efficacy equal to high-dose amoxicillin/clavulanate in a clinical trial evaluating children with persistent/recurrent AOM.

The newer regimens of azithromycin showed clinical cure rates of ~82% for AOM, despite *in vitro* data suggesting that azithromycin is still expected to cover only 25% of PNSP-R, 65% of PNSP-I, and 50% of *H influenzae*.

Additional concerns with azithromycin are higher likelihood of selecting PNSP-R with azithromycin than high-dose amoxicillin[46] and concern that concurrent use of ibuprofen and azithromycin may restrict azithromycin from reaching extracellular fluid and reduce its efficacy.[47] It may be a suitable first-line agent in the penicillin-allergic child.

Safety and Patient-Compliance Factors

In treating AOM unresponsive to first-line therapy, we considered the second-line therapies with the best:
- Safety (least potential for adverse effects)
- Patient-compliance characteristics (cost, palatability, and dosing schedule).

Our recommendations for second-line therapy, shown in **Figure 6.4**, are amoxicillin/clavulanate and cefdinir (or cefpodoxime on restricted formularies). Cefuroxime has shown some potential for success in treating refractory/recurrent AOM. But all data from the United States was obtained over 15 years ago, well before PNSP became prevalent and before PCV-7 was routinely used. It also has very poor palatability and marginal *H influenzae* activity. We do not recommend cefuroxime axetil unless its bitter taste can be masked by administering it in a bottle with formula or juice or adding commercial flavoring such as FLAVORx.

When using cefixime, once daily dosing is preferred and still the drug is not expected to cover PNSP-R or PNSP-I, while covering 100% of *H influenzae*.

Cefixime should also provide 100% coverage of *M catarrhalis*.

Third-Line Therapy

■ **AAP/AAFP Guideline Recommendations for Third-Line Therapy**

Ceftriaxone is the only antibiotic recommended for third-line therapy or amoxicillin/clavulanate failures.[4] This therapeutic option requires at minimum three to six IM injections or an intravenous line for 3 days. The cost can range from ~$400-$600 to complete the therapy. It is particularly burdensome and onerous to the family and child. It carries the risk of anaphylaxis (witnessed three times by one of the authors [SLB]), which should be explained to parents before administration, and with which practitioners need to be prepared to deal.

■ **Our Perspective**

Third-line therapy is indicated to treat AOM that has failed to respond to second-line therapy and includes (**Figure 6.4**):

- If amoxicillin/clavulanate was used for second-line therapy, our recommended choices for third-line therapy are:
  - Cefdinir (qd)
  - Cefpodoxime (bid)
- If the second-line therapy agent was a third-generation cephalosporin, our recommended choice is:
  - Amoxicillin/clavulanate ES 90 mg/6.4 mg/kg/d divided bid

Assuming that practitioners use amoxicillin/clavulanate as the second-line therapy, data from rural Kentucky pre–PCV-7 suggested that *H influenzae* was observed twice as frequently as was PNSP in children in whom amoxicillin/clavulanate failed.[48] Even newer data from children who have received PCV-7 and have refractory AOM showed that *H influenzae* is 2-fold more likely to be recovered than is *S pneumoniae*, with high-level PNSP accounting for <6% of pathogens. Thus the two broad-spectrum third-generation cephalosporins should provide reasonable coverage for children in whom amoxicillin/clavulanate failed. The caveat here is that if the child is highly febrile, PNSP may still be more likely than *H influenzae*. In this case, clindamycin can be added to cefdinir for more complete PNSP coverage.

Regardless of the second-line choice, an alternative at this point would be ceftriaxone. A practical approach to the "three-dose" regimen could be to use a "two-dose" regimen of ceftriaxone IM 50 mg/kg with the second dose administered 48 to 72 hours after the first dose. The MEE concentrations after a single dose of ceftriaxone at 24 and 48 hours are 39 and 19 µg/mL, respectively, which should be more than adequate coverage for any type of MEE pathogen. One author (SLB) recommends a follow-up office visit 7 to 10 days after the first dose has been administered, because the child has not responded to several earlier courses of antibiotic. A third ceftriaxone dose can be given if the AOM persists at this visit, but the likelihood that this child will require either tympanostomy tubes or tympanocentesis is quite high. A single dose of ceftriaxone may be considered for initial therapy in children who are difficult to dose with oral drugs or who experience vomiting and/or diarrhea.

Because ceftriaxone carries an extremely rare risk of severe (anaphylactic) allergic reaction, children administered this therapy must be observed in the office for 30 minutes after injection.

To decrease the discomfort of the injection[49]:

- Reconstitute the lyophilized ceftriaxone powder with 1% lidocaine.
- For children weighing between 10 and 20 kg, reconstitute to a higher (450 mg/mL) concentration to avoid the need for more than one site for the (maximum volume 2.0 mL) injection.

The side effects most frequently reported after injection of ceftriaxone in children were diarrhea (14.1%), diaper rash (5.2%), rash (4.9%), and vomiting (1.4%). Diarrhea due to ceftriaxone is usually transient (<5 days) and is more frequent in infants <12 months of age.[50]

One could consider the use of clindamycin 30 mg/kg/day divided tid (>90% efficacy for PNSP) as the sole therapy at this juncture only if the pathogen is known to be *S pneumoniae*. Despite the guidelines including clindamycin as a third-line alternative in penicillin-allergic children, we have several reservations about this option. Clindamycin has no gram-negative coverage, especially important in children who have received PCV-7. Also, in the past 20 years, it has shown effectiveness in only 7 of 10 children with persistent AOM (who each had PNSP).[28] Clindamycin is not FDA-approved for treatment of AOM in children.

Tympanocentesis to obtain MEE for culture and susceptibility testing should be considered to guide therapy and to drain the persistent MEE abscess.

Predicting Bacteriology of Refractory/Recurrent AOM From Prevalence Data

■ 1980s

A study by Harrison and colleagues in the 1980s showed a difference in the relative prevalence of the pathogens isolated by tympanocentesis from MEE of children who had received an antibiotic for AOM in the past 7 days compared with those who had not received an antibiotic for more than 30 days previously.[33] In this study, patients with recently treated AOM had:

- A higher prevalence of nontypeable *H influenzae* than *S pneumoniae*
- A higher prevalence of β-lactamase–producing organisms
- A higher prevalence of isolates with multiple organisms (93 with multiple organisms and 82 with single organisms in the recently treated otitis media [RTOM] compared with 6 isolates with multiple organisms and 83 with single organisms in the not recently treated ears)
- Recently treated AOM is more likely than untreated AOM to have PNSP-I.

■ 1990s

Those younger than 2 years of age with RTOM also had bilateral AOM more often than those who had not received antibiotic therapy recently (*P* <0.01).

The results of a study of the bacteriology of refractory AOM in the 1990s also found differences in the bacteriology of RTOM and not recently treated AOM (**Table 8.7**).[51] The notable differences in bacteriology in this study between ears recently treated and those not recently treated with antibiotics for AOM in this study were:

- PNSP-R was isolated from 30% of recently treated compared with only 2% of not recently treated ears.
- PNSP-I was isolated two times as often from recently treated ears.
- *H influenzae* was isolated less often from recently treated ears.

■ 2000s

Current data from children with persistent/recurrent AOM show that among children who have re-

TABLE 8.7 — Pathogens Recovered by Tympanocentesis in the 1990s From Children With Acute Otitis Media in Whom Treatment Failed in Past 3 Days

Pathogen Recovered	Last Antibiotic (Total Isolates)	
	≤3 d (63)	>3 d (220)
Streptococcus pneumoniae		
PSSP	37%	39%
PNSP-I	14%	7%
PNSP-R	30%	2%
Haemophilus influenzae		
β-Lactamase(−)	8%	21%
β-Lactamase(+)	8%	12%
Moraxella catarrhalis (+)	3%	11%
Streptococcus pyogenes	0%	7%
Totals	100%	99%

Abbreviations: PNSP-I, intermediate-level penicillin-nonsusceptible *Streptococcus pneumoniae*; PNSP-R, re-sistant penicillin-nonsusceptible *S pneumoniae*; PSSP, penicillin-susceptible *S pneumoniae*.

Data from: Block SL, et al. *Pediatr Infect Dis J.* 1995;14:751-759.

ceived PCV-7, *H influenzae* is 2-fold more likely than *S pneumoniae*. Also rates of PNSP and high level PNSP in these children are <20% and 6%, respectively.

Concordance Between Cure and Clinical Cure at 4 to 6 Days of Therapy

Even when an antibiotic is unsuccessful mid-therapy in eradicating the pathogen causing AOM, clinical success is expected in >50% at the end of therapy due to natural defenses that lead to spontaneous remissions (20% in *S pneumoniae*, 50% in *H influenzae*). A recent study compared clinical outcomes for Israeli children with AOM ages 3 to 24 months who underwent tympanocentesis and culture of MEE before initiation of antibiotic therapy and 72 to 96 hours after.[38] Of the 123 patients, about half (46%) had bacteriologic AOM failure midtherapy as determined by bacterial growth in the culture of MEE obtained 3 to 4 days after the start of therapy. End-of-therapy clinical cure rates for the two groups were:

- 63% in those with persistent pathogens midtherapy
- 97% in children with sterile MEE midtherapy (P <0.001).

Carlin and associates[39] similarly observed that two thirds of children with midtherapy bacterial persistence were still observed to be clinical successes at the end of therapy.

Thus clinical failure at the end of therapy is less likely with bacterial eradication at midtherapy. However, the correlation is far from absolute because clinical success can still occur at a lower rate (approximately 66%) despite persistent bacteria in MEE at midtherapy. The postulated causes for this are as follows:

- Technique related (culture of old drainage)
- Spontaneous remission by effects of the host immune response coupled with natural drainage of the abscess via a reopened eustachian tube
- A slower antibiotic action of a bacteriostatic drug[48]
- Draining the abscess twice in one week (double-tap studies).

Other Factors Affecting Treatment Outcome in Cases of Refractory/Recurrent AOM

While success can occur in up to 66% of cases despite midtherapy bacterial persistence (less frequent than the >90% success expected with bacterial eradication), another counterintuitive outcome may also occur, ie, clinical failure despite the pathogen in the MEE being susceptible to the prescribed and taken antibiotic. In a study by Harrison, isolates from 62% of patients with recently treated AOM were susceptible *in vitro* to the antibiotic that had most recently been prescribed, usually amoxicillin. Such findings indicate that in curing AOM, treatment failures may be due to factors other than antibiotic choice, including:

- Host factors
- Poor compliance
- Poor eustachian tube function
- Poor antibiotic absorption
- Concurrent viral illness
- Atypical copathogens
- Bacterial mutation
- Reinfection by a new pathogen.

Role of Tympanocentesis in Therapy for AOM

Tympanocentesis is taught in only a handful of residency programs. Furthermore, the procedure is uncomfortable for the patient and expensive compared with a trial of another oral medication. The results of culture and susceptibility testing are not available for 2 to 6 days. On the other hand, tympanocentesis effectively relieves the pain of an acutely inflamed and bulging tympanic membrane and in our opinion may have a small treatment effect in children with refractory AOM (10% to 15% increase in cure rate).

REFERENCES

1. Block SL. Management of acute otitis media in the 1990s. The decade of resistant pneumococcus. *Paediatr Drugs*. 1999;1:31-50.

2. Blumer JL. Fundamental basis for rational therapeutics in acute otitis media. *Pediatr Infect Dis J*. 1999;18:1130-1140.

3. Leibovitz E, Greenberg D, Piglansky L, et al. Recurrent acute otitis media occurring within one month from completion of antibiotic therapy: relationship to the original pathogen. *Pediatr Infect Dis J*. 2003;22:209-216.

4. American Academy of Pediatrics Subcommittee on Management of Acute Otitis Media. Diagnosis and management of acute otitis media. *Pediatrics*. 2004;113:1451-1465.

5. Block SL, Hedrick J, Harrison CJ, et al. Community-wide vaccination with the heptavalent pneumococcal conjugate significantly alters the microbiology of acute otitis media. *Pediatr Infect Dis J*. 2004;23:829-833.

6. Casey JR, Pichichero ME. Changes in frequency and pathogens causing acute otitis media in 1995-2003. *Pediatr Infect Dis J*. 2004;23:824-828.

7. Block SL, Busman TA, Paris MM, Bukofzer S. Comparison of five-day cefdinir treatment with ten-day low dose amoxicillin/clavulanate treatment for acute otitis media. *Pediatr Infect Dis J*. 2004;23:834-838.

8. Black S, Shinefield H, Fireman B, et al. Efficacy, safety and immunogenicity of heptavalent pneumococcal conjugate vaccine in children. Northern California Kaiser Permanente Vaccine Study Center Group. *Pediatr Infect Dis J*. 2000;19: 187-195.

9. Black S, Shinefield H, Baxter R, et al. Postlicensure surveillance for pneumococcal invasive disease after use of heptavalent pneumococcal conjugate vaccine in Northern California Kaiser Permanente. *Pediatr Infect Dis J*. 2004;23:485-489.

10. Eskola J, Kilpi T, Palmu A, et al. Efficacy of a pneumococcal conjugate vaccine against acute otitis media. *N Engl J Med*. 2001;344:403-409.

8

11. Block SL, Harrison CJ, Hedrick J, Tyler R, Smith A, Hedrick R. Restricted use of antibiotic prophylaxis for recurrent acute otitis media in the era of penicillin non-susceptible *Streptococcus pneumoniae*. *Int J Pediatr Otorhinolaryngol*. 2001;61:47-60.

12. Block, SL, Hedrick JA, Harrison CJ. Widespread use of conjugated pneumococcal vaccine significantly reduces rates of AOM and antibiotic usage. 2004 Pediatric Academic Societies' Annual Meeting; San Francisco, Calif; May 1-4, 2004. Abstract #1135.

13. Poehling KA, Lafleur BJ, Szilagyi PG, et al. Population-based impact of pneumococcal conjugate vaccine in young children. *Pediatrics*. 2004;114:755-761.

14. McEllistrem MC, Adams J, Mason EO, Wald ER. Epidemiology of acute otitis media caused by *Streptococcus pneumoniae* before and after licensure of the 7-valent pneumococcal protein conjugate vaccine. *J Infect Dis*. 2003;188:1679-1684.

15. Dagan R, Givon-Lavi N, Zamir O, et al. Reduction of nasopharyngeal carriage of Streptococcus pneumoniae after administration of a 9-valent pneumococcal conjugate vaccine to toddlers attending day care centers. *J Infect Dis*. 2002;185:927-936.

16. Bogaert D, van Belkum A, Sluijter M, et al. Colonisation by *Streptococcus pneumoniae* and *Staphylococcus aureus* in healthy children. *Lancet*. 2004;363:1871-1872.

17. Fireman B, Black SB, Shinefield HR, Lee J, Lewis E, Ray P. Impact of the pneumococcal conjugate vaccine on otitis media. *Pediatr Infect Dis J*. 2003;22:10-16.

18. Jones VF, Harrison CJ, Stout GG, Hopkins J. Nasopharyngeal colonization with heptavalent pneumococcal conjugate vaccine serotypes of *Streptococcus pneumoniae* with prolonged vaccine dosing intervals. *Pediatr Infect Dis J*. 2005. In press.

19. Caspary H, Welch JC, Lawson L, et al. Impact of pneumococcal polysaccharide vaccine (Prevnar) on middle ear fluid in children undergoing tympanostomy tube insertion. *Laryngoscope*. 2004;114:975-980.

20. Harrison CJ, Welch DF. Middle ear effusion amoxicillin concentrations in acute otitis media. *Pediatr Infect Dis J.* 1998;17:657-658.

21. Seikel K, Shelton S, McCracken GH. Middle ear fluid concentrations of amoxicillin after large dosages in children with acute otitis media. *Pediatr Infect Dis J.* 1997;16:710-711.

22. Canafax DM, Yuan Z, Chonmaitree T, Deka K, Russlie HQ, Giebink GS. Amoxicillin middle ear fluid penetration and pharmacokinetics in children with acute otitis media. *Pediatr Infect Dis J.* 1998;17:149-156.

23. Block SL, McCarty JM, Hedrick JA, Nemeth MA, Keyserling CH, Tack KJ and the Cefdinir Otitis Media Study Group. Comparative safety and efficacy of cefdinir vs amoxicillin/clavulanate for treatment of suppurative acute otitis media in children. *Pediatr Infect Dis J.* 2000;19(suppl 12):S159-S165.

24. Block SL, Kratzer J, Nemeth MA, Tack KJ. Five-day cefdinir course vs ten-day cefprozil course for treatment of acute otitis media. *Pediatr Infect Dis J.* 2000;19(suppl 12):S147-S152.

25. Dagan R, Hoberman A, Johnson C, et al. Bacteriologic and clinical efficacy of high dose amoxicillin/clavulanate in children with acute otitis media. *Pediatr Infect Dis J.* 2001;20:829-837.

26. Block SL, Hedrick JA, Kratzer J, Nemeth MA, Tack KJ. Five-day twice daily cefdinir therapy for acute otitis media: microbiologic and clinical efficacy. *Pediatr Infect Dis J.* 2000;19(suppl 12):S153-S158.

27. Bottenfield GW, Burch DJ, Hedrick JA, Schaten R, Rowinski CA, Davies JT. Safety and tolerability of a new formulation (90 mg/kg/day divided every 12 hr of amoxicillin/clavulanate (Augmentin) in the empiric treatment of pediatric acute otitis media caused by drug-resistant *Streptococcus pneumoniae. Pediatr Infect Dis J.* 1998;17:963-968.

28. Jorgensen JH, Doern GV, Maher LA, Howell AW, Redding JS. Antimicrobial resistance among respiratory isolates of *Haemophilus influenzae, Moraxella catarrhalis,* and *Streptococcus pneumoniae* in the United States. *Antimicrob Agents Chemother.* 1990;34:2075-2080.

8

29. Schwartz RH, Rodriguez WJ, Khan WN. Persistent purulent otitis media. *Clin Pediatr*. 1981;20:445-447.

30. Block SL, Harrison CJ, Hedrick JA, et al. Penicillin-resistant *Streptococcus pneumoniae* in acute otitis media: risk factors, susceptibility patterns and antimicrobial management. *Pediatr Infect Dis* J. 1995;14:751-759.

31. Barry B, Gehanno P, Blumen M, Boucot I. Clinical outcome of acute otitis media caused by pneumococci with decreased susceptibility to penicillin. *Scand J Infect Dis*. 1994;26:446-452.

32. del Castillo F, Baquero-Artigao F, Garcia-Perea A. Influence of recent antibiotic therapy on antimicrobial resistance of *Streptococcus pneumoniae* in children with acute otitis media in Spain. *Pediatr Infect Dis J*. 1998;17:94-97.

33. Harrison CJ, Marks MI, Welch DF. Microbiology of recently treated acute otitis media compared with previously untreated acute otitis media. *Pediatr Infect Dis J*. 1985;4:641-646.

34. Pichichero ME. Recurrent and persistent otitis media. *Pediatr Infect Dis J*. 2000;19:911-916.

35. Jacobs MR. Optimisation of antimicrobial therapy using pharmacokinetic and pharmacodynamic parameters. *Clin Microbiol Infect*. 2001;7:589-596.

36. Pelton S. Acute otitis media. In: Long SS, Pickering LK, Prober CG, eds. *Principles and Practice of Pediatric Infectious Diseases*. 2nd ed. Philadelphia, Pa: Churchill Livingstone; 2002.

37. Howie VM, Dillard R, Lawrence B. In vivo sensitivity test in otitis media: efficacy of antibiotics. *Pediatrics*. 1985;75:8-13.

38. Dagan R, Leibovitz E, Leiberman A, Yagupsky P. Clinical significance of antibiotic resistance in acute otitis media and implication of antibiotic treatment on carriage and spread of resistant organisms. *Pediatr Infect Dis J*. 2000;19(suppl 5):S57-S65.

39. Carlin SA, Marchant CD, Shurin PA, Johnson CE, Super DM, Rehmus JM. Host factors and early therapeutic response in acute otitis media. *J Pediatr*. 1991;118:178-183.

40. Marchant CD, Carlin SA, Johnson CE, Shurin PA. Measuring the comparative efficacy of antibacterial agents for acute otitis media: the 'Pollyanna phenomenon'. *J Pediatr.* 1992; 120:72-77.

41. Craig WA, Andes D. Pharmacokinetics and pharmacodynamics of antibiotics in otitis media. *Pediatr Infect Dis J.* 1996;15:255-259.

42. Harrison CJ. Using antibiotic concentrations in middle ear fluid to predict potential clinical efficacy. *Pediatr Infect Dis J.* 1997;16(suppl 2):S12-S16.

43. Block SL. Causative pathogens, antibiotic resistance and therapeutic considerations in acute otitis media. *Pediatr Infect Dis J.* 1997;16:449-456.

44. Block SL, Arrieta A, Seibel M, McLinn S, Eppes S, Murphy MJ. Single-dose (30 mg/kg) azithromycin compared with 10-day amoxicillin/clavulanate for the treatment of uncomplicated acute otitis media: a double-blind, placebo-controlled, randomized clinical trial. *Curr Ther Res Clin Exp.* 2003; 64(suppl A):A30-A42.

45. Arrieta A, Arguedas A, Fernandez P, et al. High-dose azithromycin versus high-dose amoxicillin-clavulanate for treatment of children with recurrent or persistent acute otitis media. *Antimicrob Agents Chemother.* 2003;47:3179-3186.

46. Samore MH, Magill MK, Alder SC, et al. High rates of multiple antibiotic resistance in *Streptococcus pneumoniae* from healthy children living in isolated rural communities: association with cephalosporin use and intrafamilial transmission. *Pediatrics.* 2001;108:856-865.

47. Mandell GL, Coleman EJ. Effect of antipyretic agents on uptake, transport, and release of antimicrobial agents by human polymorphonuclear leukocytes. *J Infect Dis.* 2002;185: 1314-1319.

48. Block SL, Hedrick JA, Tyler RD, Smith RA, Harrison CJ. Microbiology of acute otitis media recently treated with aminopenicillins. *Pediatr Infect Dis J.* 2001;20:1017-1021.

8

49. Bradley JS. Oral vs. intramuscular antibiotic therapy for acute otitis media: which is best? *Pediatr Infect Dis J*. 1999;18:1147-1151.

50. Harrison CJ, Welch D, Marks MI. Ceftriaxone therapy in pediatric patients. *Am J Dis Child*. 1983;137:1048-1051.

51. Dagan R, Leibovitz E, Greenberg D, Yagupsky P, Fliss DM, Leiberman A. Early eradication of pathogens from middle ear fluid during antibiotic treatment of acute otitis media is associated with improved clinical outcome. *Pediatr Infect Dis J*. 1998;17:776-782.

9

Tympanostomy Tubes

Tympanostomy tubes are used to manage conductive hearing loss associated with middle ear effusion (MEE) and for prevention of recurrent acute otitis media (AOM). Various reports have estimated that from 500,000[1] to >1 million[2] tympanostomy tubes are placed in the United States each year.

A large recent meta-analysis[3] called into question the long-term benefits of placement of pressure-equalizing (PE) tubes for persistent otitis media with effusion (OME) unless underlying developmental or genetic conditions exist. No real difference in detectable advantages was found in otherwise well children as to cognitive or developmental parameters, despite a rapid normalization of hearing when PE tubes are in place.

Criteria for When to Insert Tympanostomy Tubes

Indications for tympanostomy tube insertion include[4-7]:

- Treatment of AOM refractory to three or four sequential courses of different efficacious antimicrobials and/or three daily intramuscular injections of ceftriaxone
- Treatment of bilateral persistent MEE (chronic OME) lasting >4 to 6 months[4,5]
- Prevention of recurrent AOM after five to six well-documented episodes of AOM in 1 year separated by intervals of documented normal tympanic function
- Prevention of recurrent AOM after four episodes of AOM during the summer or fall in healthy children 6 to 18 months old

- Prevention of recurrent AOM after three episodes of AOM in infants <6 months old or those with prior history of significant hearing loss
- Prevention of AOM after several episodes of AOM in those with Down syndrome or cleft palate
- Human immunodeficiency virus (HIV)–infected hosts with more than three episodes of AOM in 1 year
- To manage retraction pocket or hypertrophic white sclerosis that might develop into a cholesteatoma
- To manage acute mastoiditis or intracranial AOM complications.

When these criteria for insertion of tubes were used, rates of 5% to 8% for insertion of PE tubes in the first 24 months have been observed recently in rural Kentucky. These are similar to those published from Pittsburgh and New England.

Laser-Assisted Tympanostomy

Increased availability of laser-assisted insertion of tympanostomy tubes may result in this technology being used as an adjunct to tube placement in some cases,[6] but the cost of the instrument and lack of enthusiasm in the overall medical community have prevented its widespread use.

Care of Tympanostomy Tubes

The major concerns in caring for a child who has had tympanostomy tubes inserted are to avoid introducing external ear canal flora as pathogens into the middle ear through the tube and to monitor for possible complications.

■ Water Exposure

There is a small risk that activities such as swimming and bathing will lead to water entering the middle ear through an intact tympanostomy tube. Therefore, patients with tubes are usually advised to use fitted ear plugs during activities that could result in water entering the external canal.[2] For patients who have suffered persistent or recurrent drainage from PE tubes, water avoidance in the ears is prudent when bathing or swimming.

■ Physician Follow-Up Care After Surgery

The child with tympanostomy tubes should initially be seen by a physician after surgery to check that the tubes are functional. Otolaryngologists recommend a follow-up visit between 2 and 4 weeks after tube insertion for evaluation of the results of surgery by[2]:

- Otomicroscopic examination to verify proper position and function of the tube and resolution of retraction pocket or other structural abnormalities for which surgery was indicated
- Audiometry (ideally in a soundproof room) to document hearing and the benefits of surgery if there was hearing loss due to MEE preoperatively.

Most episodes of tube otorrhea can be managed by a primary care provider. Otolaryngologists surveyed recently estimated that only about 4% of the 75,000 children they treated in the previous year had a complication with tympanostomy tubes that might have been avoided by earlier referral to the specialist.

For most children, tubes may be electively removed if they have failed to extrude after an average of 2.5 years.[7]

■ Reopening a Blocked Tube

A blocked tube may be reopened by administering ototopical antibiotic drops or lavage with hydrogen peroxide for 5 to 7 days. Suspensions designed for otic use or solutions designed for ophthalmic use (gentamicin) are less acidic and therefore less irritating to middle ear mucosa than hydrogen peroxide. Some otic solutions may contain ethylene glycol or alcohol and induce burning pain when used with patent PE tubes. If the patient tastes the drops or complains of stinging when hydrogen peroxide is used, it is probably because the liquid has reached the nasopharynx through an unclogged tympanostomy tube.

A skilled practitioner may be able to unclog some plastic tympanostomy tubes using a 3-French metal suction catheter under otomicroscopic guidance.[2]

Otorrhea and Tympanostomy Tubes

Nonpurulent otorrhea can be a normal sequela of tympanostomy tube placement in the 2 weeks following placement. Purulent otorrhea is a sign that the ear is infected.[2]

■ Otorrhea as a Normal Sequela of Tympanostomy Tube Placement

When evaluating the implications of otorrhea with tympanostomy tube placement, it is important to remember[2]:

- Up to 10% of children have serous discharge from the ear in the first 2 weeks after tympanostomy tube placement, regardless of surgical technique, ear canal preparation, or use of antibiotic otic drops. This is likely due to overactive mucous secretory goblet cells stimulated by long-term low oxygen tension in the middle ear. This should subside as the goblet cells readjust to normal gas content.

- A later-onset episode of purulent otorrhea may be expected within 6 months in one half of children after tympanostomy tube placement.

■ Otorrhea as a Sign of AOM

When a young child develops acute otorrhea (<1-week duration) through a tympanostomy tube in association with an upper respiratory tract infection, it is likely that the pathogen is one typical of AOM (ie, *Streptococcus pneumoniae, Haemophilus influenzae, Moraxella catarrhalis,* or group A Streptococcus), and antibiotic therapy is recommended.

Systemic (oral) administration of antibiotics with or without a topical antibiotic may be used. Our recommendation is for oral antibiotic therapy with the choice of the agent being based on the relative local prevalence of pathogens and antibiotic resistance. Topical ofloxacin alone has shown success in treating infection in these cases.

Recent data suggest that in nonfebrile children with recent-onset otorrhea, addition of a steroid to the quinolone shortens the time to cessation of drainage, and may even reduce granulation tissue.[8] Granulation tissue is one of the main causes of recurrent and chronic otorrhea in children with PE tubes in place. These children typically respond well to antibiotics, but the condition recurs rapidly after stopping antibiotics. Most require tube removal and debridement for resolution. If the ciprofloxacin plus dexamethasone reduced granulation tissue enough, perhaps some tubes could be salvaged. Our experience has been that prolonged (> 3 weeks) use of quinolone-steroid drops appears to increase the chance of *Candida* or methicillin-resistant *Staphylococcus aureus* (MRSA) superinfection. So if otorrhea persists beyond 10 days of steroid combination topical otic therapy, otolaryngologic referral is warranted for debridement and culture from the tube orifice.

We have reported that about 50% of pathogens recovered are penicillin-nonsusceptible *S pneumoniae* (PNSP) strains in this scenario. Antibiotics with more activity against intermediate PNSP (PNSP-I) should be selected initially. Therefore, culture from the os of the tube may be worthwhile.

For refractory cases of otorrhea, instilling topical antibiotics after ear toileting (suctioning of debris) from the external canal every day enhances resolution of otorrhea.

Otorrhea for >2 weeks is more likely to be due to pathogens other than standard AOM pathogens. They usually include bacteria found in the external ear canal (eg, *Pseudomonas, Proteus*), MRSA, or even candida species. In these cases, cultures of drainage directly from the PE tube opening are important. Culture of drainage from the canal is likely to reveal external ear flora, which may or may not be causing the otorrhea.

If *Candida albicans* is isolated from chronic otorrhea, we have had ~70% success using fluconazole (4-6 mg/kg/day dosed once daily) oral therapy for 10 to 14 days. Cessation of any steroid-containing topicals is also important. MRSA is quite difficult to eradicate from PE tubes associated with otorrhea[9] and intravenous vancomycin has been advocated. Susceptibilities dictate the choice of potential antibiotic systemic therapy. When there are susceptibilities, we have found success with oral therapy to equal that of intravenous therapy.

Successful 3-week regimens include:

- A combination of trimethoprim-sulfamethoxazole (10 mg/kg/day divided every 12 hours) plus rifampin (this requires a pharmacy to formulate it as a liquid at 20 mg/kg/day divided every 12 hours)

- Clindamycin 30 mg/kg/day divided every 8 hours (ensure that the D-test is negative), and linezolid.

The latter is very expensive and is used mostly by subspecialists. If otorrhea does not improve dramatically within 5 days, otolaryngologic referral is needed. The increased prevalence of MRSA otorrhea mirrors the increased MRSA in soft tissue and skin infections occurring throughout the United States. One recent study suggests that this may be due to universal pneumococcal conjugate vaccine (PCV)–7 immunization eradicating the competing pneumococcal strains in the nasopharynx.[10]

Risks of Tympanostomy Tubes

Risks of tympanostomy tubes include risks of the procedure for tube placement and risks of complications of therapy.

■ Risks of the Procedure for Tube Placement
Risks of the procedure to place tympanostomy tubes include:
- Risk of death due to general anesthesia (approximately 1/40,000 children)[11]
- Risk of sensorineural hearing loss due to damage to the round window during tube placement (the risk of this complication can be eliminated by not placing tubes in the posteroinferior quadrant).[12]

■ Other Complications of Tympanostomy Tube Therapy in Addition to Otorrhea
Possible complications of tympanostomy tube therapy include:
- Increased risk of tympanosclerosis (1.4% excess risk[7])

- Formation of granulation tissue (probably due to ongoing inflammation) (2.2% risk[7]). This tissue can be the nidus that causes recurrent or persisting otorrhea despite proper antibiotic therapy
- Migration of the tube into the middle ear (0.2% risk[7])
- Permanent perforation of the tympanic membrane (TM), with risk being related to tube type (0% to 4% for short-term tubes and 12% to 25% for long-term tubes[2])
- Weakening of the TM, increasing the risk of future perforation (1.7% risk[6]) and formation of a retraction pocket[2]
- Development of cholesteatoma in a deep retraction pocket or behind the eardrum (0.4% risk[7]; this does not include the risk of tympanostomy tube placement performed to treat retraction pocket or cholesteatoma).

Retraction pocket (pouching of the TM into the middle ear) can occur as a complication of chronic OME and as such may be treated by tympanostomy tube placement. *Cholesteatoma* (overgrowth of epithelial cells within a retraction pocket or in the middle ear space after a chronic TM perforation) can occur as a complication of tympanostomy tube therapy. The effects on hearing of possible complications of tympanostomy tube placement probably depend on the type of complication and its effect on the vibratory capacity of the TM. For example, tympanosclerosis has been reported to cause negligible hearing loss,[2] but an air-bone gap of more than 40 dB can occur when there is significant intratympanic involvement.[13]

In response to a society survey,[7] otolaryngologists reported an overall complication rate (including recurrent AOM) of 17% in approximately 75,000 children undergoing tympanostomy tube placement over the course of the previous year. The most frequent complications were:

- Recurrent or persistent otorrhea (78 per 1000 cases)
- Retention of tube for >2 years (27/1000 cases)
- Granulation tissue or foreign-body reaction (22/1000 cases)
- Atelectasis (18/1000 cases)
- Perforation of the TM after extrusion of the tube (17/1000 cases)
- Excessive tympanosclerosis (14/1000 cases)
- Cholesteatoma (4/1000 cases).

Cost of Tympanostomy Tube Therapy

The cost of therapy is now being considered in weighing the relative benefits and risks of alternatives for treatment. The total cost of tympanostomy tube placement in the United States has been estimated at a minimum of $1200 per procedure.[14] When tympanostomy tube placement is indicated for managing chronic OME, managed-care health insurers may require a trial of antibiotic prophylaxis (approximate cost for antibiotics and follow-up visits, $400) and documentation that the trial failed before approving surgery.[11] However, we advise against this practice[6] because the resolution of OME with antibiotic therapy is <10% and the antibiotic burden will increase resistance during a time when we are trying to limit antibiotic use.

If PCV-7 reduces PE tube use by 20% as reported in the Kaiser-Permanente Study,[15] cost savings could be large. For example, 100,000 less PE tube surgeries per year could save $2.4 billion or more per year.

Efficacy of Tympanostomy Tubes

The success of tympanostomy tubes in treating and preventing recurrent AOM has been compared with placebo (no other treatment) or, for preventing AOM, with antibiotic prophylaxis.

■ Compared With Placebo

According to Isaacson and Rosenfeld, several large studies have shown that tympanostomy tubes are superior to placebo in managing OME and recurrent AOM in selected groups.[2]

■ Compared With Antibiotic Prophylaxis

New research shows that the efficacy of antibiotic prophylaxis has decreased because of increasing resistance of AOM pathogens to these drugs. Therefore, tympanostomy tubes may now be superior to antibiotic prophylaxis in preventing recurrent AOM.

REFERENCES

1. Block SL. Management of acute otitis media in the 1990s: the decade of resistant pneumococcus. *Paediatr Drugs.* 1999;1:31-50.

2. Isaacson G, Rosenfeld RM. Care of the child with tympanostomy tubes. *Pediatr Clin North Am.* 1996;43:1183-1193.

3. Lous J, Burton M, Felding J, Ovesen T, Rovers M, Williamson I. Grommets (ventilation tubes) for hearing loss associated with otitis media with effusion in children. *Cochrane Database Syst Rev.* 2005;(1):CD001801.

4. Paradise JL, Feldman HM, Campbell TF, et al. Effect of early or delayed insertion of tympanostomy tubes for persistent otitis media on developmental outcomes at the age of three years. *N Engl J Med.* 2001;344:1179-1187.

5. Shriberg LD, Friel-Patti S, Flipsen P, Brown RL. Otitis media, fluctuant hearing loss, and speech-language outcomes: a preliminary structural equation model. *J Speech Lang Hear Res.* 2000;43:100-120.

6. Morris MS. Tympanostomy tubes: types, indications, techniques, and complications. *Otolaryngol Clin North Am.* 1999;32:385-390.

7. Derkay CS, Carron JD, Wiatrak BJ, Choi SS, Jones JE. Postsurgical follow-up of children with tympanostomy tubes: results of the American Academy of Otolaryngology—Head and Neck Surgery Pediatric Otolaryngology Committee National Survey. *Otolaryngol Head Neck Surg.* 2000;122:313-318.

8. Roland PS, Dohar JE, Lanier BJ, et al; CIPRODEX AOMT Study Group. Topical ciprofloxacin/dexamethasone otic suspension is superior to ofloxacin otic solution in the treatment of granulation tissue in children with acute otitis media with otorrhea through tympanostomy tubes. *Otolaryngol Head Neck Surg.* 2004;130:736-741.

9. Hartnick CJ, Shott S, Willging JP, Myer CM 3rd. Methicillin-resistant *Staphylococcus aureus* otorrhea after tympanostomy tube placement: an emerging concern. *Arch Otolaryngol Head Neck Surg.* 2000;126:1440-1443.

10. Bogaert D, van Belkum A, Sluijter M, et al. Colonisation by *Streptococcus pneumoniae* and *Staphylococcus aureus* in healthy children. *Lancet.* 2004;363:1871-1872.

11. Block SL. Commentary. *Pediatric Infections Forum.* 2000;2:4-5, 13.

12. Rosenfeld RM. Natural history of untreated otitis media. In: Rosenfeld RM, Bluestone CD, eds. *Evidence-Based Otitis Media.* St. Louis Mo: BC Decker, Inc; 1999:157-177.

13. Asiri S, Hasham A, Ul Anazy F, Zakzouk S, Banjar A. Tympanosclerosis: review of literature and incidence among patients with middle-ear infection. *J Laryngol Otol.* 1999;113:1076-1080.

14. Dowell SF, Marcy SM, Phillips WR, Gerber MA, Schwartz B. Otitis media – principles of judicious use of antimicrobial agents. *Pediatrics.* 1998;101(suppl):165-171.

15. Black S, Shinefield H, Fireman B, et al. Efficacy, safety and immunogenicity of heptavalent pneumococcal conjugate vaccine in children. Northern California Kaiser Permanente Vaccine Study Center Group. *Pediatr Infect Dis J.* 2000;19:187-195.

9

10 Complications

The functions of the ear are hearing and balance. Acute otitis media (AOM) is almost always complicated by a reversible mild to moderate conductive hearing loss in the affected ear, due to the presence of middle ear effusion (MEE). Because a sterile (noninfected) MEE (otitis media with effusion [OME]) persisting for up to 3 months is an expected complication of successfully treated AOM, mild conductive hearing loss is also to be expected for several weeks after an episode of AOM. Other common complications of treated or untreated AOM are persistent/recurrent AOM and perforation of the tympanic membrane (TM), with or without secondary external otitis. Possible complications of AOM are shown in **Figure 10.1**.[1]

Uncommonly, more serious and even life-threatening complications have been documented after AOM.

Anatomy of Local and Contiguous Structures

Figure 10.2 shows a diagram of the middle ear and surrounding structures and the location of common and uncommon complications of AOM.

Expected Complications of AOM

Minor complications that are so common they are almost expected to occur after an episode of AOM include:

- OME and transient conductive hearing loss
- Persistent/recurrent AOM

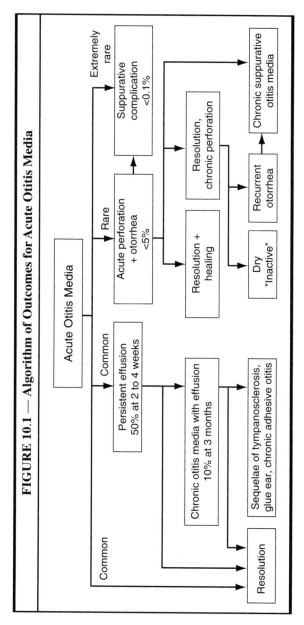

FIGURE 10.1 — Algorithm of Outcomes for Acute Otitis Media

FIGURE 10.2 — Possible Complications of Acute Otitis Media

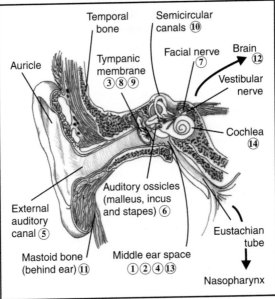

1. Temporary (to 1 month) conductive hearing loss
2. Otitis media with effusion (OME)
3. Acute perforation of tympanic membrane (TM)
4. Persistent/recurrent acute otitis media (AOM)
5. Extrusion of tympanostomy tubes
6. Discontinuity of ossicles
7. Facial nerve paralysis
8. Chronic perforation of the TM
9. Tympanosclerosis
10. Vertigo
11. Mastoiditis
12. Meningitis
13. Cholesteatoma
14. Permanent sensorineural hearing loss

10

- Perforation of the TM, acute or with secondary external otitis.

■ Otitis Media With Effusion and Conductive Hearing Loss

OME (sterile MEE) is a common occurrence after resolution of AOM. The MEE resolves in about half of cases within 1 month of the infection, but about 10% of children will still have MEE up to 3 months after resolution of AOM.[1]

MEE causes conductive hearing loss mostly in high frequency ranges, usually between 15 and 40 dB and not >60 dB, when the fluid occupies sufficient middle ear space to dampen sound transmission. Hearing usually returns to normal after the MEE has resolved. However, conductive hearing loss may rarely become permanent after recurrent AOM or chronic OME or ossicular discontinuity or fixation.[2]

The rationale for treating persistent MEE and non-infectious complications of AOM is that hearing forms the neurophysiologic foundation for the development of language and cognition. This foundation is established in the first 3 years of life, coincident with the highest risk of MEE. As a result, physicians and caregivers often feel a sense of urgency to minimize the severity and duration of hearing loss due to MEE during this critical period.

Analysis of the literature through the early 1990s reveals no consistent, reliable evidence that otherwise healthy children 1 to 3 years old suffer any long-term effects when hearing loss of ≤20 dB occurs bilaterally for <4 months.[3] A more recent study found that in otherwise healthy children <2 years of age, total or bilateral MEE (estimated from diagnoses at health care visits) is weakly correlated with a negative impact on vocabulary, as rated by parents using the MacArthur Communicative Development Inventory-Words and Sentences tool.[4] In another recent study, children 24 to 60 months old with OME had reduced scores on the gross motor portion of the Peabody Developmental Motor Scales before tympanostomy tube placement, but after surgery their scores exceeded scores of children without OME.[5]

Using a different approach, Paradise and colleagues examined the relationship between parental stress and children's behavior problems in the first 3 years of life with the duration of MEE. They found that stress, as rated by parents, was inversely related to socioeconomic status but had no relationship to duration of MEE. Behavior problems in youngsters with MEE are associated with socioeconomic status and not MEE.[6] Roberts and associates also studied environmental effects and found that both OME and hearing loss were more strongly related to the quality of home and child-care environments than to children's language and cognitive development. They suggest that children in less responsive caregiving environments experience conditions more conducive to OME (eg, smoking). Also, it may be more difficult for caregivers to continue to be responsive and stimulating with children who have more OME.[7]

To evaluate the potential for PE placement to reduce developmental and/or speech and language delay caused by OME and its accompanying hearing loss, Paradise and colleagues additionally followed 6350 infants. Of these, 400 had sufficient OME to cause further evaluation with developmental and language assessments. Half were randomized to receive PE tubes at the usual 3 to 4 months of effusion, and half received PE tubes up to 9 months later. By 3 years of age, no differences were detected in the verbal or cognitive abilities or in receptive language, sentence length, grammar complexity, or behavior. This suggests that there is no rush to place PE tubes for OME. One could justify waiting 6 months into OME with hearing loss to refer for PE tube placement, unless that individual patient showed delay in speech or had other contributing issues, such as a preexisting neurologic problem or Down syndrome.[8]

Placement of tympanostomy tubes appears to provide real but mainly short-term benefits:

- Rapid restoration of hearing that persists as long as functioning tubes are in place (mean 3 to 9 months).
- Reduction in the number of episodes of AOM (averaging one to three less episodes per year)
- Maintenance of development, as much potential as is possible, in children at risk for developmental problems, eg, Down syndrome, children with visual impairment, birth injuries.

These benefits come at a fair cost, and usually requires general anesthesia. The potential adverse outcomes are uncommon and usually reversible. The most recent large meta-analysis in a Cochrane report[9] reemphasized these issues and suggested that tube placement for OME was not justified without bilateral hearing loss of >20 db. This brings up the issue of just how to measure such hearing losses in infants and young children without resorting to very expensive techniques, such as brain stem–evoked-response testing.

Future research is needed to pinpoint what permanent deficits result from specific degrees of hearing loss at specific times during development. The recommendation for otherwise healthy children 1 to 3 years old with MEE after AOM is that when OME has persisted for more than 4 months, accompanied by a bilateral loss of $\geq$20 dB, tympanostomy tube placement should be considered. The incidence of OME is higher in young children. For example, in a group of 86 African-American children in day care[10]:

- 70% of children had bilateral OME >35% of the time between ages 6 and 24 months

- Only 13% experienced bilateral OME for >35% of the time between ages 24 and 60 months.

Uncommon and Less Serious Complications of AOM

Uncommon, less serious complications of AOM can be acute or chronic.

■ Less Serious Complications of Acute Otitis Media
Acute/Uncommon
An early uncommon, less serious complication of AOM is extrusion of tympanostomy tubes.

Chronic/Uncommon
Chronic uncommon, less serious complications of AOM include chronic perforation of the TM, adhesive otitis, and tympanosclerosis.

Uncommon, Serious Complications of AOM

Since the advent of antibiotics, serious complications of AOM are so uncommon that many primary care practitioners never see them. They include:
- Vertigo
- Temporal bone osteitis (Gradenigo's syndrome)
- Mastoiditis
- Cholesteatoma
- Meningitis
- Sigmoid sinus thrombosis (estimated incidence of 0.002% of AOM episodes)
- Otitic hydrocephalus
- Facial nerve paralysis (estimated incidence of 0.005% of AOM episodes).

Among 100 children hospitalized between 1980 and 1995 in Pittsburgh with an intratemporal complication of AOM[11]:

- 72% had acute mastoiditis; of those, 54 (75%) were treated with broad-spectrum intravenous antibiotics and myringotomy and 18 (25%) required mastoidectomy
- 22% had facial paralysis; of those, 18 (82%) were treated conservatively but four required mastoid surgery
- 3% with serous labyrinthitis recovered completely with conservative therapy, but 2% with suppurative labyrinthitis had permanent profound sensorineural hearing loss in the affected ear
- 4% had acute petrositis that resolved with mastoidectomy in all cases.

In a recent report,[12] five of seven children with venous sinus thrombosis had one or more coagulation abnormalities, pointing out the need to evaluate such children for prothrombotic disorders, eg, factor V Leiden mutations or elevated lipoprotein apoprotein.

■ Mastoiditis

Recently, there has been increased interest in acute mastoiditis as a complication of AOM. Bahadori and colleagues reported a nearly 3-fold increase in acute mastoiditis in Northern Virginia in the era of drug-resistant *Streptococcus pneumoniae*, ie, from 1991 through 1999.[13] A parallel increase noted by Ghaffar and associates in the 1990s in Texas[14] was confirmed by a more recent report by Zapalac and colleagues.[15] The Ghaffar group reported that many of these children did not have a history of frequent AOM. Zapalac and associates noted that two thirds of the pneumococcal isolates from their patients were resistant to penicillin. In contrast, Kaplan and colleagues reported a stable rate of mastoiditis during the same period in a multicenter study despite increasing rates of antibiotic-resistant *S pneumoniae*.[16] They also reported that serogroup 19 (included in the pneumococcal conjugate vaccine [PCV]) was the leading cause of pneumococcal mastoiditis.

Mastoiditis is another arena in which PCV could have a marked impact. Because most investigators felt that drug-resistant pneumococcus played a role in the increase in mastoiditis and other intracranial complications of AOM, universal use of the vaccine could have positive effects. First, it could reduce the amount of disease due to serotype 19F, which was noted by Kaplan and colleagues to be the most common cause of mastoiditis. Second, most penicillin-nonsusceptible *S pneumoniae* (PNSP) organisms are included in the seven serotypes found in the conjugate vaccine,[17] so reductions in drug resistance produced by the vaccine would improve the likelihood that the usual antibiotics used to treat AOM would restrict spread of this pathogen to the mastoid and temporal bone.

Of course, recent data indicate PCV-7 offers as much as 56% protection against AOM due to serotype 6B but as little as 19% for 19F, so that the vaccine may have less impact than desired. Pneumococcal serotype 19A is also emerging as PCV-7 serotypes diminish, and it is as drug resistant as 19F, so we may not see less mastoiditis from PCV-7 use, despite the end of vaccine shortages. Further, group A streptococcus and *Staphylococcus aureus* are becoming more prominent in acute mastoiditis,[18] particularly when it occurs in children that are not otitis prone. These may be the reasons for continued reports of increased prevalence of acute mastoiditis.[19]

It will be interesting to see if the increased trend in mastoiditis seen in the late 1990s will reverse throughout the next decade now that the vaccine is universally advocated in young children.

223

■ Vertigo

Vertigo due to labyrinthitis may be caused by increased tension of the round-window membrane. Or it might occur by spread of infection from the middle ear through the mastoid or petrous bone intracranially to cause inflammations of the 7th or 8th cranial nerve, which may then extend extracranially into the labyrinth. Labyrinthitis is associated with temporary or permanent sensorineural hearing loss.

■ Cholesteatoma

Cholesteatoma is an uncommon but serious complication of AOM. Cholesteatoma may be treated by tympanostomy tube placement, but it may also occur as a complication of tympanostomy tube placement done to manage recurrent AOM or persistent OME. It may accompany persistent otorrhea, particularly malodorous otorrhea.

■ Meningitis

Meningitis is a preventable but rare sequela of severe AOM. Other intracranial complications of AOM that have been documented in children and adults include[20]:

- Dural sinus thrombosis due to spread of inflammation from the mastoid
- Extradural or epidural abscess (usually composed of granulation tissue rather than pus) is most often due to destruction of bone adjacent to the dura by cholesteatoma or chronic suppurative otitis media
- Subdural empyema, a collection of purulent material between the dura and arachnoid membrane, usually develops after AOM by direct extension of infection
- Brain abscess may be caused by AOM (extremely rarely), acute mastoiditis (rarely), or another complication of AOM.

■ Other

Extremely rare complications include discontinuity of middle ear ossicles and facial nerve paralysis.

REFERENCES

1. Dowell SF, Marcy SM, Phillips WR, Gerber MA, Schwartz B. Otitis media – principles of judicious use of antimicrobial agents. *Pediatrics.* 1998;101(suppl):165-171.

2. Bluestone CD. Epidemiology and pathogenesis of chronic suppurative otitis media: implications for prevention and treatment. *Int J Pediatr Otorhinolaryngol.* 1998;42:207-223.

3. Otitis Media Guideline Panel. Managing otitis media with effusion in young children. *Pediatrics.* 1994;94:766-773.

4. Feldman HM, Dollaghan CA, Campbell TF, et al. Parent-reported language and communication skills at one and two years of age in relation to otitis media in the first two years of life. *Pediatrics.* 1999;104:e52.

5. Orlin MN, Effgen SK, Handler SD. Effect of otitis media with effusion on gross motor ability in preschool-aged children: preliminary findings. *Pediatrics.* 1977;99:334-337.

6. Paradise JL, Feldman HM, Colborn DK, et al. Parental stress and parent-rated child behavior in relation to otitis media in the first three years of life. *Pediatrics.* 1999;104:1264-1273.

7. Roberts JE, Burchinal MR, Zeisel SA, et al. Otitis media, the caregiving environment, and language and cognitive outcomes at 2 years. *Pediatrics.* 1998;102:346-354.

8. Paradise JL, Feldman HM, Campbell TF, et al. Effect of early or delayed insertion of tympanostomy tubes for persistent otitis media on developmental outcomes at the age of three years. *N Engl J Med.* 2001;344:1179-1187.

9. Lous J, Burton M, Felding J, Ovesen T, Rovers M, Williamson I. Grommets (ventilation tubes) for hearing loss associated with otitis media with effusion in children. *Cochrane Database Syst Rev.* 2005;(1):CD001801.

10

10. Zeisel SA, Roberts JE, Neebe EC, Riggins R Jr, Henderson FW. A longitudinal study of otitis media with effusion among 2- to 5-year-old African-American children in child care. *Pediatrics.* 1999;103:15-19.

11. Goldstein NA, Casselbrant ML, Bluestone CD, Kurs-Lasky M. Intratemporal complications of acute otitis media in infants and children. *Otolaryngol Head Neck Surg.* 1998;119: 444-454.

12. Oestreicher-Kedem Y, Raveh E, Kornreich L, Yaniv I, Tamary H. Prothrombotic factors in children with otitis media and sinus thrombosis. *Laryngoscope.* 2004;114:90-95.

13. Bahadori RS, Schwartz RH, Ziai M. Acute mastoiditis in children: an increase in frequency in Northern Virginia. *Pediatr Infect Dis J.* 2000;19:212-215.

14. Ghaffar FA, Wordemann M, McCracken GH. Acute mastoiditis in children: a seventeen-year experience in Dallas, Texas. *Pediatr Infect Dis J.* 2001;20:376-380.

15. Zapalac JS, Billings KR, Schwade ND, Roland PS. Suppurative complications of acute otitis media in the era of antibiotic resistance. *Arch Otolaryngol Head Neck Surg.* 2002;128:660-663.

16. Kaplan SL, Mason EO, Wald ER, et al. Pneumococcal mastoiditis in children. *Pediatrics.* 2000;106:695-699.

17. Harrison CH, Stout GG, Buck G, Jones F. Serotype proportions relative to pneumococcal conjugate vaccine (PCV) types and antibiotic resistance in *Streptococcus pneumoniae* (Spn) in Louisville, KY. Abstract #1606. PAS Baltimore, Md; May, 2002.

18. Migirov L, Kronenberg J. Bacteriology of mastoid subperiosteal abscess in children. *Acta Otolaryngol.* 2004;124:23-25.

19. Robinson RF, Koranyi K, Mahan JD, Nahata MC. Increased frequency of acute mastoiditis in children. *Am J Health Syst Pharm.* 2004;61:304, 306.

20. Rosenfeld RM. Natural history of untreated otitis media. In: Rosenfeld RM, Bluestone CD, eds. *Evidence-Based Otitis Media.* St. Louis, Mo: BC Decker, Inc; 1999:157-177.

11 Prevention

Using knowledge gained from pathophysiologic, epidemiologic, and pharmacologic studies of acute otitis media (AOM), clinicians and researchers have evaluated numerous methods to decrease the burden of AOM on children, their families, the health care system, and society. Measures proposed to address eustachian tube (ET) dysfunction, prevent viral upper respiratory infection (URI), and prevent infection with bacterial pathogens of AOM include surgical procedures, environmental measures, chemoprophylaxis, and vaccination against predisposing viruses and bacterial pathogens.

Surgical Procedures to Prevent Recurrent AOM

Children with persistent and recurrent AOM almost universally have ET dysfunction. Pressure equalizing (PE) tubes are effective because they allow air to enter the middle ear space by bypassing the ET, thereby allowing air flow from the external canal. Because of their risks, surgical procedures are a last resort to decrease the risk of recurrent AOM in patients who have AOM refractory to four or more courses of antibiotics or multiple episodes of clustered recurrent AOM. Surgical procedures that have been investigated for their usefulness in preventing recurrent AOM and associated middle ear effusion (MEE) lasting up to a month or more include:

- Myringotomy (incision of the tympanic membrane [TM]) or tympanocentesis (puncture of the TM with removal of MEE for sampling) is effective in relieving pain due to an existing episode of AOM. However, the TM opening closes within 2 to 5 days, preventing any durable effect on MEE and AOM.

- The use of tympanostomy tubes to decrease the risk of recurrent AOM was discussed in Chapter 9, *Tympanostomy Tubes*. The overall effectiveness of tympanostomy tube placement in preventing recurrent episodes of AOM or persistent otitis media with effusion (OME) is quite high (~70% to 80%).[1] However, these effects on OME are only sure to be present as long as the tubes are present. If the ETs have not matured sufficiently, the effusions of OME may return quickly. A recent meta-analysis (Cochrane report) on efficacy of tympanostomy tubes emphasized that long-term benefits of PE tube placement for OME have not been demonstrated in otherwise normal hosts, so delaying placement until a >20 dB hearing loss is documented for >4 months is justified.[2]

- Laser myringotomy (LM) alone was not as effective as tympanostomy tube placement via scalpel myringotomy or LM in a small Polish study with ~30 subjects per group; there were 36% recurrences with LM alone and 11% with myringotomy plus tubes.[3]

- Instead of tympanostomy tubes, Finnish investigators evaluated adenoidectomy with or without once-daily sulfisoxazole antibiotic prophylaxis (50 mg/kg/day) vs no intervention and found no reduction in AOM episodes, physician visits, or antibiotic use overall.[4] Their conclusion was that adenoidectomy is not as effective as tympanostomy tubes as initial surgical intervention for recurrent AOM.

- Adenoidectomy significantly decreases the risk of recurrent AOM in otitis-prone children who continue to have OME or recurrent AOM with tympanostomy tubes in place or after extrusion of a prior set of tubes.[5] We recommend concurrent adenoidectomy if and when a second set of tympanostomy tubes is indicated. In a recent review, Bluestone estimated that the average rate of adenoidectomy for this indication is about 1.2%.[6]

- In addition to the need for pneumococcal vaccine and consideration of antibiotic prophylaxis, a new recommendation for tympanostomy tube placement has arisen for those children receiving cochlear implants for severe sensorineural hearing deficits. Children who have more than two AOM episodes in 4 months or more than three in 6 months should have tubes placed until they outgrow their otitis-prone condition[7] to reduce AOM episodes that threaten the integrity of the implants and raise the chance of invasive pneumococcal central nervous system infection.

Environmental Measures to Prevent AOM

11

Environmental measures help prevent AOM by decreasing the risks of ET inflammation and/or URI. Significant benefits have been identified for the following measures:
- Decreasing contact with persons who have URI (mainly, avoidance of day care)
- Avoiding exposure to tobacco smoke
- Breast-feeding rather than bottle-feeding for the first 12 months of life
- Avoiding bottle propping
- Shifting from bottle-feeding as soon as feasible
- Minimizing use of pacifiers.

As discussed in Chapter 2, *Epidemiology*, and Chapter 3, *Pathophysiology, Immunology, and Natural History*, viral URI is a major risk factor for AOM. In addition, children from families with atopy are at significantly higher risk of AOM compared with their cohorts in day care, particularly when they are exposed to sources of allergens such as pets or a carpet or rug (see next section). Because of these indirect associations between atopy and higher risk of AOM, avoiding allergens is believed to decrease the risk of AOM primarily in older children.

■ Decreasing Exposure to Upper Respiratory Tract Pathogens

More than 60% of children in the United States attend some form of day care,[8] and day care attendance, particularly by those <2 years of age, is one of the more significant risk factors for URI and AOM.[9] For children with a family history of atopy, day care attendance in the first year of life more than doubles the risk of two or more physician-diagnosed ear infections (relative risk [RR] 2.4), sinusitis (RR 2.2), or lower respiratory illness (RR 1.6), and the risk is even higher when day care involves exposure to pets, a carpet or rug, or is provided in a day care facility (more children) rather than a home (fewer children).[8]

A study by Niemela and colleagues found that children in day care who use a pacifier are at somewhat greater increased risk (RR 1.6) for an episode of AOM compared with those in day care who do not use pacifiers regularly (only for sleep or stress), and that the younger the child, the greater the risk.[10] In this study, those <2 years of age in day care who used a pacifier had 5.4 episodes of AOM per year compared with 3.6 for those in day care who did not use a pacifier. For children 2 to 3 years old in day care who used a pacifier, the incidence of AOM increased from 1.9 to 2.7 episodes a year.[10]

In summary, measures to decrease the risks of AOM due to day care include:

- Decreasing time in day care
- Using day care with fewer children
- Avoiding pacifier use by children in day care
- Avoiding exposure to allergens for children with a personal or family history of atopy.

A child's risk of AOM is also directly related to and increases with higher number of siblings in the household.

■ Breast-feeding

Breast-feeding rather than bottle-feeding for at least the first 3 months of life has been associated with decreased risk of AOM.[11] The risk of AOM increases gradually after discontinuation of breast-feeding, with longer duration of breast-feeding conferring a longer period of decreased risk (up to 12 months) after discontinuation.[12] Human milk contains immunoglobulins and numerous antipathogenic substances[12] that may act by oligosaccharide binding to active sites on pathogens, including *Streptococcus pneumoniae*, preventing their attachment to cell walls.[5]

■ Exposure to Tobacco Smoke

Exposure to tobacco smoke irritates the respiratory tract, promoting the inflammatory changes in the ET that can lead to development of MEE and increased risk of AOM. Adderson reviewed the relationship between so-called passive smoking and AOM and found that the relationship was inconsistent in earlier studies relying exclusively on parental history as an indication of exposure to tobacco smoke. However, there was a clear relationship between parental smoking and increased risk of otitis media in four studies that carefully controlled for confounding variables or that measured children's serum or urine concentrations of cotinine (a nicotine metabolite).[11] For example, one of these later studies showed that among children attending a day care center, those with a serum cotinine concentration of 2.5 ng/mL or higher had a 38% higher rate of new episodes of MEE and otitis media episodes (AOM or OME) of longer duration.[13]

Chemoprophylaxis

Pharmacologic agents that have shown efficacy in decreasing the incidence of AOM include antibiotics and xylitol.

■ Antibiotic Prophylaxis

In the 1970s and 1980s (before the widespread prevalence of penicillin-nonsusceptible *S pneumoniae* [PNSP]), low-dose amoxicillin (20 mg/kg/d) had a reasonable rate of success in preventing AOM. Up to 3 months of chemoprophylaxis (daily low dose) with sulfisoxazole or amoxicillin was common to prevent recurrent AOM in otitis-prone children. One meta-analysis found that this chemoprophylaxis regimen prevented about one episode of AOM annually in otitis-prone children.[14] A more recent meta-analysis calculated that it prevented about 0.25 episode/patient-month in populations at higher risk and 0.06 episode/patient-month in populations at lower risk of recurrent AOM.[15] Thus the overall benefit of chemoprophylaxis was relatively small but the risks and cost were also small compared with those of tympanostomy tube insertion.

However, the potential benefits of antibiotic prophylaxis for AOM are now overshadowed by the rapid increase in incidence of antibiotic-resistant pathogens. For example, Mandel and colleagues found in a study performed in 1990 to 1992 that 20 mg/kg/d amoxicillin was significantly ($P <0.001$) more effective than placebo in preventing new episodes of AOM and MEE.[16] However, Roark and Berman reported that 20 mg/kg/d amoxicillin during the era of PNSP (1993 to 1994), whether administered in a single dose or two divided doses, was no more successful than placebo in preventing new episodes of AOM in otitis-prone children 3 months to 6 years of age.[17] But the diagnostic criteria used for AOM in this study might have allowed inclusion of OME, which does not require therapy with antibiotics.

Antibiotic prophylaxis may not prove successful in preventing recurrent AOM and it probably increases rates of resistant pathogens. Continuous daily prophylaxis has also been shown to be more effective than intermittent prophylaxis at the onset of URI.

Some experts feel there still may be a role for chemoprophylaxis. When antibiotic prophylaxis is selected, clinicians should follow these guidelines to increase the possible benefit and decrease the risk of promoting further development of antibiotic-resistant strains of AOM pathogens[1]:

- Limit prescriptions to children who have four or more episodes of AOM within 6 months.
- Avoid prescribing broader-spectrum antimicrobials (eg, cephalosporins or amoxicillin/clavulanate) for prophylaxis.
- Limit duration of prophylaxis to about 4 to 6 weeks.

11

■ Xylitol Prophylaxis

Xylitol prophylaxis for AOM has been investigated in Europe and may prove useful if problems with dosing and side effects can be overcome. Xylitol is a five-carbon sugar with an alcohol moiety that is added as a sweetener to food, chewing gum, and toothpaste and inhibits growth of *Streptococcus mutans* and *S pneumoniae in vitro*. It was formulated as a syrup to test its effectiveness in decreasing the risk of AOM in very young children. In healthy young children in out-of-home day care, five doses of xylitol syrup a day

233

for 3 months reduced the incidence of AOM significantly, from about three episodes to about two episodes per year.[18]

Problems with xylitol prophylaxis include the high likelihood of noncompliance with multiple daily doses, the possible gastrointestinal and other side effects that the 8.4-g dose studied would have in infants,[19] and the fact that the possible adverse effects of long-term therapy are unknown. Compared with a cost of $3500 for office visits and antibiotic treatment for four episodes of AOM followed by insertion of tympanostomy tubes in 6% to 8% of the young population, xylitol could be administered for 3 months at a cost of only $378. Although this option is less costly than antibiotic prophylaxis or tympanostomy tube placement, its efficacy in general practice has yet to be confirmed. A recent preliminary report indicated that xylitol does not reduce AOM if given only when the child has new upper respiratory infection symptoms.[20]

Viral Immunization

Effective antiviral immunoglobulins and vaccines have been developed for passive or active immunization against viral URIs that can predispose to AOM.

■ Passive Immunization

Balancing efficacy against risk, immunoprophylaxis with polyclonal RSV-IV-Ig (RespiGam) or palivizumab (Synagis) is only indicated to decrease the risk of respiratory compromise due to respiratory syncytial virus (RSV) infection in those at high risk for severe complications of lower respiratory tract infection, such as:

- Children <2 years with bronchopulmonary dysplasia requiring oxygen therapy
- Those infants in their first RSV season after being born at <32 weeks gestation.

In such patients, prevention of AOM is only a beneficial side effect and not an indication for RSV-Ig-IV immunoprophylaxis. RSV prophylaxis with RSV-Ig-IV has been superceded for routine cases by the use of Synagis intramuscularly.

■ Active Immunization

Vaccination against influenza has proven effective in decreasing influenza illness in healthy children by 10% to 40% in the year of administration and in decreasing the incidence of AOM during and soon after influenza season. The reduction in AOM risk through prevention of influenza is particularly important because influenza seems to promote AOM in three ways: it causes mucosal inflammation leading to ET dysfunction; it directly facilitates colonization by *S pneumoniae* in both children and adults; and children may become infected with two different influenza strains within one winter season. Influenza vaccination is recommended or suggested for persons at high risk for serious disease or complications of influenza, or anyone wishing to avoid influenza-induced disease.

Trivalent (Intramuscular) Influenza Vaccine

The currently licensed influenza vaccine, a trivalent inactivated vaccine (TIV) that contains three formalin-killed strains (H1N1, H3N2, and B) that may vary annually, is administered intramuscularly (IM). One study documents that vaccination with TIV decreases the risk of AOM.[21] While this vaccine is not recommended for children <6 months, it may benefit children >6 months of age who are at high risk for AOM. It is also recommended for caregivers to prevent spread of infection.

For children 6 months to 13 years old, influenza immunization with the purified surface antigen "split-virus" formulation of TIV is recommended, because this formulation carries lower risk of adverse reactions

235

than the whole-cell vaccine. A child's first-ever influenza vaccination (at <9 years of age) should be administered as two IM doses at least 1 month apart. For subsequent annual vaccinations, a single injection is usually effective. The vaccine is updated by manufacturers annually by cocultivation with that year's wild-type A and B master strains.

Cold-Adapted (Intranasal) Influenza Vaccine

In a recent study by Belshe and colleagues,[22] an intranasal spray form of influenza vaccine was well tolerated and effective in preventing influenza in healthy children 15 to 71 months old who were administered one dose (89% efficacy) or two doses 1 month apart (94% efficacy). Overall, vaccinated children had 30% fewer episodes of "febrile otitis media" compared with the control group.[22] But diagnostic criteria for AOM were not given (possibly included both OME and AOM). Termed cold-adapted influenza vaccine (CAIV), the intranasal formulation is genetically altered to grow at temperatures found in human nasal cavities (about 32°C) but not in internal organs such as the lung (37°C or higher).

Children in the first study who continued for year 2 (85%) received a single dose of CAIV (0.5 mL, administered as a 0.25-mL spray into each nostril). This single dose proved 92% efficacious in preventing culture-confirmed influenza and 33% effective in preventing otitis media for which antibiotic therapy would have been prescribed.[23]

As of the spring of 2005, CAIV (Flumist) was approved for otherwise healthy individuals 5 to 49 years of age. Ongoing international studies of younger children may allow approval by the Food and Drug Administration (FDA) for 6-month to 5-year-olds by late 2005 or 2006. Concerns that it might provoke bronchospasm in asthma patients in part prompted the additional studies.

There are also new and encouraging data on phase 2 evaluation of live attenuated parainfluenza type 3 (PIV3)–cold passage mutant 45 (cp45) vaccine which was conducted in 380 children 6 to 18 months old to prevent croup. Parainfluenza is a common antecedent to AOM. This vaccine was safe, immunogenic, and did not in itself provoke AOM in the immediate follow-up period over a rate seen with placebo recipients.[24] Only further studies will show whether it reduces later AOM episodes during "croup season." Additionally, RSV and parainfluenza construct vaccines using fusion proteins are in clinical trials.

Bacterial (Pneumoccocal) Immunization

Techniques have been sought for pediatric immunization against *S pneumoniae* (pneumococcus) because this organism accounts for most invasive bacterial infections in young children in the United States. Colonization of the nasopharynx by *S pneumoniae*, which can lead to AOM, pneumonia, or bacteremia, can be detected in infancy and peaks toward the second to third year of life.[25]

There are at least 90 different serotypes of *S pneumoniae*, but only about two dozen cause significant pneumococcal disease. Furthermore, nine serotypes cause 90% of pneumococcal infections in children,[26] and meta-analysis of a number of studies showed that only seven serotypes (3, 4, 6B, 14, 18C, 19F, and 23F) were identified in almost 80% of cases of AOM in which *S pneumoniae* was isolated.[27] Thus efforts to develop a pneumococcal vaccine effective in decreasing the incidence of AOM have focused on providing immunity against the currently most common AOM serotypes for children at highest risk for AOM (those <2 years old). Most PNSP are included in serotypes of PCV-7 (>85%), so universal use of pneumococcal conjugate vaccine (PCV)–7 in infants may reduce AOM but is even more likely to reduce AOM due to PNSP. Based on AOM isolates from the mid 1990s, we expect a larger effect on younger children because 7- to 24-month old children have nearly 3-fold more AOM due to vaccine serotypes (**Figure 11.1** and **Table 11.1**). Likewise, younger children have more drug resistance that correlates with vaccine serotypes. The FDA-approved PCV-7 vaccine for active immunization against serotypes causing AOM has been moderately successful, more so than originally predicted (see below).

■ Passive Immunization

When high serum antibody titers are achieved, passive immunization with bacterial polysaccharide immunoglobulin (BPIG) can temporarily decrease the risk of AOM due to *S pneumoniae* types covered by the vaccine. However, the effect was studied only in children at high risk for AOM, was limited to the serotypes included, and was short-lived.[27]

■ Active Immunization

A 23-valent purified polysaccharide pneumococcal vaccine for IM or subcutaneous injection has been available for a number of years. According to a review by Adderson, adverse effects of this vaccine (severe local reaction, fever, myalgia, allergic reaction) are rare and it may be administered with other vaccines.[11] However, it has limited effectiveness in immunocompromised patients and it has not been found effective in children younger than 24 months except in one study that indicated efficacy in an African-American population.[28]

A recent meta-analysis of all pneumococcal vaccine studies showed that 23-valent polysaccharide vaccine had a modest effect in reducing AOM but only when used in children who were both >24 months of age and otitis prone.[29] Another study showed that

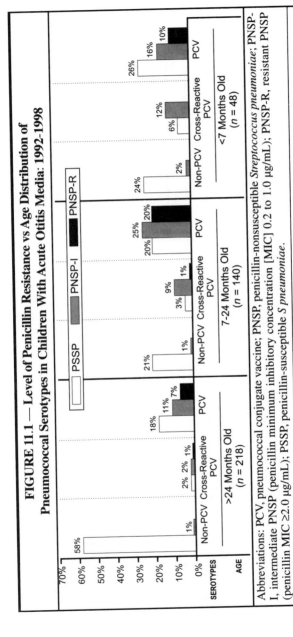

FIGURE 11.1 – Level of Penicillin Resistance vs Age Distribution of Pneumococcal Serotypes in Children With Acute Otitis Media: 1992-1998

Abbreviations: PCV, pneumococcal conjugate vaccine; PNSP, penicillin-nonsusceptible *Streptococcus pneumoniae*; PNSP-I, intermediate PNSP (penicillin minimum inhibitory concentration [MIC] 0.2 to 1.0 µg/mL); PNSP-R, resistant PNSP (penicillin MIC ≥2.0 µg/mL); PSSP, penicillin-susceptible *S pneumoniae*.

Adapted from: Block SL, et al. *Pediatr Infect Dis J*. 2002;21:859-865.

11

TABLE 11.1 — Decreasing Proportion of _Streptococcus pneumoniae_ and Increased Nontypeable _Haemophilus influenzae_ in AOM After Community-Wide Use of Pneumococcal Conjugate Heptavalent Vaccine

Pathogen	% AOM Pathogens From Pre–PCV-7 Era (1992-1998) n = 336	% AOM Pathogens From Post–PCV-7 (2000-2003) n = 83
PSSP	23	12
PNSP-I	16	13
PNSP-R	9	6
All SP	**48**	**31**
ntHi (-)	18	20
ntHi (+)	23	36
All ntHi	**41**	**56**
Mcat (+)	9	11
GAS	2	2

Abbreviations: AOM, acute otitis media; GAS, group A streptococcus; Mcat, *Moraxella catarrhalis*; MIC, minimum inhibitory concentration; ntHi (-), β-lactamase–negative nontypeable *H influenzae*; ntHi (+), β-lactamase–positive nontypeable *H influenzae*; PNSP-I, penicillin-nonsusceptible *S pneumoniae*–intermediate (MIC 0.1–1.0 mg/L); PNSP-R, penicillin-nonsusceptible *S pneumoniae*–resistant (MIC ≥2.0 mg/L); PSSP, penicillin-susceptible *S pneumoniae* (MIC <0.1 mg/L); PCV-7, pneumococcal conjugate heptavalent vaccine.

Larger drop in proportion of penicillin-susceptible than in penicillin-resistant pneumococci (23% to 12% vs 25% to 19%). Annualized rate of AOM requiring tympanocentesis also dropped from 48 to 23 cases per year.

Block SL, et al. *Pediatr Infect Dis J.* 2004;23:829-833.

11

PCV-7 strains were not eliminated by use of the 23-valent pneumococcal vaccine as a booster to a single PCV-7 dose both given in the second year of life, however 2 doses of PCV-7 did reduce PCV-7 strains. Interestingly, serotypes not in PCV-7 completely replaced the PCV-7 strains, so that overall pneumococcal colonization rates were not changed regardless of which or how many doses of vaccine were used.[30]

Conjugated polysaccharide-protein vaccines are more immunogenic in young infants,[13] and randomized controlled trials of a heptavalent PCV (Prevnar) were completed. The trials showed PCV to be safe and effective in children younger than 2 years for preventing invasive disease by S pneumoniae from serotypes in the vaccine (4, 6B, 9V, 14, 18C, 19F, and 23F). In June 2000, the American Academy of Pediatrics (AAP) Committee on Infectious Diseases recommended adding PCV to the pediatric immunization schedule. The 2000 AAP recommendations for vaccination of previously unvaccinated children are shown in **Table 11.2**.[31]

The serotypes from which the PCV-7 vaccine polysaccharides were derived represented 70% to 80% of middle ear isolates from children in the United States,[18] so widespread pneumococcal immunization of children <2 years in the United States with PCV-7 according to the recommended schedule was projected to result in a modest reduction in the incidence of AOM due to S pneumoniae. In one early study, children who received PCV-7 made only 9% fewer visits to the physician for AOM but had a 20% lower rate of tympanostomy tube insertion compared with those not receiving the vaccine.[32] However, the reduction in incidence of AOM was 43% for otitis-prone children after the fourth dose. Even with the decrease that had been expected to be <10% in cases of AOM, it seemed reasonable to use the PCV, particularly in previously unimmunized patients >24 months old in day care with

TABLE 11.2 — Recommended Schedule of Doses for Pneumococcal Immunization (PCV) in Previously Unvaccinated Children*

Risk Level	Age at First Dose	Primary Series	Booster Dose
Any	2 to 6 months	3 doses, 6 to 8 weeks apart	1 dose at 12 to 15 months of age
Any	7 to 11 months	2 doses, 6 to 8 weeks apart	1 dose at 12 to 15 months of age
Any	12 to 23 months	2 doses, 6 to 8 weeks apart	—
High	24 months or older	1 dose	—

Abbreviation: PCV, heptavalent pneumococcal polysaccharide-protein conjugated vaccine.

* If vaccine is fully available. Modifications in these recommendations arise when shortages of vaccine occur.

Centers for Disease Control and Prevention. Recommended Childhood Immunization Schedule—United States, 2001. *MMWR Morb Mortal Wkly Rep.* 2001;50:7-18.

11

recurrent AOM or past history of PE tubes who might not otherwise fit criteria of the AAP for vaccination.[30]

Despite on-and-off vaccine shortages, the result of universal infant PCV-7 use has been a somewhat better than expected decrease in overall AOM rates, particularly recalcitrant AOM, plus pneumococcal serotype substitution. Serotype substitution is a shift away from PCV-7 serotypes and toward nonvaccine serotypes with one benefit being less overall antibiotic-resistant pneumococci causing AOM (more PCV-7 strains are highly penicillin resistant than nonvaccine strains). The other change has been an overall increase in nontypeable *Haemophilus influenzae* in AOM, particularly in AOM in which initial amoxicillin therapy has failed. These changes have improved the utility of drugs with excellent activity against β-lactamase–producing *H influenzae*, eg, the second- and third-generation cephalosporins that are β-lactamase stable (cefdinir, cefuroxime axetil, cefpodoxime proxetil, and even cefixime). The use of these drugs in recurrent or persistent AOM had been hindered by their lack of activity against penicillin-nonsusceptible *S pneumoniae* (PNSP) with minimum inhibitory concentrations (MICs) >0.5 mg/L. Now that the absolute number of these strains has decreased due to PCV-7, clinicians can use these drugs with increased confidence as second-line AOM drugs (**Table 11**.3). This sentiment was reinforced in the recent AAP/American Academy of Family Physicians (AAFP) guideline for treating uncomplicated AOM (spring 2004) (see Chapter 8, *Second-Line and Third-Line Antibiotic Therapy* for more details).

■ **Immunization Against Other Bacterial Pathogens**

Although studies have been conducted in animals to identify antibodies against nontypeable *H influenzae* that might be useful in a vaccine, there are

244

many strains, and the antibodies against one serotype do not necessarily cross-protect against others.[27]

REFERENCES

1. Block SL. Commentary. *Pediatric Infections Forum.* 2000;2: 4-5, 13.

2. Lous J, Burton M, Felding J, Ovesen T, Rovers M, Williamson I. Grommets (ventilation tubes) for hearing loss associated with otitis media with effusion in children. *Cochrane Database Syst Rev.* 2005;(1):CD001801.

3. Hassmann E, Skotnicka B, Baczek M, Piszcz M. Laser myringotomy in otitis media with effusion: long-term follow-up. *Eur Arch Otorhinolaryngol.* 2004;261:316-320.

4. Koivunen P, Uhari M, Luotonen J, et al. Adenoidectomy versus chemoprophylaxis and placebo for recurrent acute otitis media in children aged under 2 years: randomised controlled trial. *BMJ.* 2004;328:487.

5. Klein JO. Nonimmune strategies for prevention of otitis media. *Pediatr Infect Dis J.* 2000;19(suppl 5):S89-S92.

6. Bluestone CD. Pathogenesis of otitis media: role of eustachian tube. *Pediatr Infect Dis J.* 1996;15:281-291.

7. Luntz M, Teszler CB, Shpak T. Cochlear implantation in children with otitis media: second stage of a long-term prospective study. *Int J Pediatr Otorhinolaryngol.* 2004;68:273-280.

8. Celedon JC, Litonjua AA, Weiss ST, Gold DR. Day care attendance in the first year of life and illnesses of the upper and lower respiratory tract in children with a familial history of atopy. *Pediatrics.* 1999;104:495-500.

9. Sipila M, Karma P, Pukander J, Timonen M, Kataja M. The Bayesian approach to the evaluation of risk factors in acute and recurrent acute otitis media. *Acta Otolaryngol.* 1988;106:94-101.

11

TABLE 11.3 — Expected Clinical Failures Based on Proportions of AOM Pathogens Isolated at Tympanocentesis From Kentucky Children Pre–PCV-7 (1992-1998) and Post–PCV-7 (2000-2003)

Drug	Dosage	Pre–PCV-7 (1992-1998) (%)	Post–PCV-7 (2000-2003) (%)
Amoxicillin	45 mg/kg/day	27	27
Amoxicillin	90 mg/kg/day	14	19
Amoxicillin/clavulanate	45 mg/kg/day	17	12
Amoxicillin/clavulanate	90 mg/kg/day	5	4
Azithromycin	10 mg/kg × 3 days	29	27
Azithromycin	30 mg/kg × 1 dose	23	24
Cefdinir	14 mg/kg/day	16	10
Cefuroxime axetil	30 mg/kg/day	19	13
Cefpodoxime proxetil	10 mg/kg/day	18	13
Cefixime	8 mg/kg/day	23	15
Cefprozil	30 mg/kg/day	30	29

Clindamycin	30 mg/kg/day	23	29
Trimethoprim/sulfamethoxazole	10/50 mg/kg/day divided q12h	35	24

Abbreviations: AOM, acute otitis media; Mcat, *Moraxella catarrhalis*; ntHi, nontypeable *Haemophilus influenzae*; PNSP-I, penicillin-nonsusceptible *Streptococcus pneumoniae*–intermediate; PNSP-R, penicillin-nonsusceptible *S pneumoniae*–resistant; PSSP, penicillin-susceptible *S pneumoniae*; PCV-7, pneumococcal conjugate heptavalent vaccine.

Pathogens in AOM, 1992-1998: 15% sterile, 40% pneumococcus (17% PSSP, 14% PNSP-I, 9% PNSP-R), 36% nontypeable *H influenzae* (ntHi: 20% β-lactamase producers, 16% nonproducers), 9% *Moraxella catarrhalis* (Mcat: all β-lactamase producers). Pathogens in AOM, 2000-2003: 15% sterile, 26% pneumococcus (11% PSSP, 11% PNSP-I, 4% PNSP-R), 53% ntHi (33% β-lactamase producers, 20% nonproducers, 5% Mcat). Calculations assume spontaneous remission in 20% of pneumococci and 50% of *haemophilus* and *moraxella*.

11

10. Niemela M, Uhari M, Mottonen M. A pacifier increases the risk of recurrent acute otitis media in children in day care centers. *Pediatrics.* 1995;96:884-888.

11. Adderson EE. Preventing otitis media: medical approaches. *Pediatr Ann.* 1998;27:101-107.

12. Sassen ML, Brand R, Grote JJ. Breast-feeding and acute otitis media. *Am J Otolaryngol.* 1994;15:351-357.

13. Etzel RA, Pattishall EN, Haley NJ, Fletcher RH, Henderson FW. Passive smoking and middle-ear effusion among children in day care. *Pediatrics.* 1992;90:228-232.

14. Williams RL, Chalmers TC, Stange KC, Chalmers FT, Bowlin SJ. Use of antibiotics in preventing recurrent acute otitis media and in treating otitis media with effusion. A meta-analytic attempt to resolve the brouhaha. *JAMA.* 1993;270:1344-1351.

15. Rosenfeld RM. What to expect from medical treatment of otitis media. *Pediatr Infect Dis J.* 1995;14:731-738.

16. Mandel EM, Casselbrant ML, Rockette HE, Bluestone CD, Kurs-Lasky M. Efficacy of antimicrobial prophylaxis for recurrent middle ear effusion. *Pediatr Infect Dis J.* 1996;15:1074-1082.

17. Roark R, Berman S. Continuous twice daily or once daily amoxicillin prophylaxis compared with placebo for children with recurrent acute otitis media. *Pediatr Infect Dis J.* 1997;16:376-381.

18. Uhari M, Kontiokari T, Niemela M. A novel use of xylitol sugar in preventing acute otitis media. *Pediatrics.* 1998;102:879-884.

19. Mitchell AA. Xylitol prophylaxis for acute otitis media: tout de suite? *Pediatrics.* 1998;102:974-975.

20. Tapiainen T, Luotonen L, Kontiokari T, Renko M, Uhari M. Xylitol administered only during respiratory infections failed to prevent acute otitis media. *Pediatrics.* 2002;109:E19.

21. Clements DA, Langdon L, Bland C, Walter E. Influenza A vaccine decreases the incidence of acute otitis media in 6- to 30-month-old children in day care. *Arch Pediatr Adolesc Med*. 1995;149:1113-1117.

22. Belshe RB, Mendelman PM, Treanor J, et al. The efficacy of live attenuated, cold-adapted, trivalent, intranasal influenzavirus vaccine in children. *N Engl J Med*. 1998;338:1405-1412.

23. Belshe RB, Gruber WC. Prevention of otitis media in children with live attenuated influenza vaccine given intranasally. *Pediatr Infect Dis J*. 2000;19(suppl 5):S66-S71.

24. Belshe RB, Newman FK, Tsai TF, et al. Phase 2 evaluation of parainfluenza type 3 cold passage mutant 45 live attenuated vaccine in healthy children 6-18 months old. *J Infect Dis*. 2004;189:462-470.

25. Dagan R, Fraser D. Conjugate pneumococcal vaccine and antibiotic-resistant *Streptococcus pneumoniae*:herd immunity and reduction of otitis morbidity. *Pediatr Infect Dis J*. 2000;19(suppl 5):S79-S88.

26. Giebink GS. Vaccination against middle-ear bacterial and viral pathogens. *Ann NY Acad Sci*. 1997;830:330-352.

27. Pelton SI, Klein JO. The promise of immunoprophylaxis for prevention of acute otitis media. *Pediatr Infect Dis J*. 1999;18:926-935.

28. Howie VM, Ploussard JH. Efficacy of fixed combination antibiotics versus separate components in otitis media. Effectiveness of erythromycin estrolate, triple sulfonamide, ampicillin, erythromycin estolate-triple sulfonamide, and placebo in 280 patients with acute otitis media under two and one-half years of age. *Clin Pediatr*. 1972;11:205-214.

29. Straetemans M, Sanders EA, Veenhoven RH, Schilder AG, Damoiseaux RA, Zielhuis GA. Review of randomized controlled trials on pneumococcal vaccination for prevention of otitis media. *Pediatr Infect Dis J*. 2003;22:515-524.

30. Veenhoven RH, Bogaert D, Schilder AG, et al. Nasopha-ryngeal pneumococcal carriage after combined pneumo-coccal conjugate and polysaccharide vaccination in children with a history of recurrent acute otitis media. *Clin Infect Dis.* 2004;39:911-919.

31. American Academy of Pediatrics Committee on Infec-tious Diseases. Policy Statement: Recommendations for the Prevention of Pneumococcal Infections, Including the Use of Pneumococcal Conjugated Vaccine (Prevnar), Pneumococcal Polysaccharide Vaccine, and Antibiotic Prophylaxis. Issued June 5, 2000. http://www.aap.org/policy/re9960.html.

32. Black S, Shinefield H, Fireman B, et al. Efficacy, safety and immunogenicity of heptavalent pneumococcal con-jugate vaccine in children. Northern California Kaiser Permanente Vaccine Study Center Group. *Pediatr Infect Dis J.* 2000;19:187-195.

12 Case Presentations

The following sample cases illustrate how to select antibiotic therapy for acute otitis media (AOM) in various presentations.

■ Case 1: Development of Pneumonia in Afebrile Child With AOM

Pneumonia develops in an afebrile 3-year-old patient with AOM refractory to amoxicillin. Up to half of cases of community-acquired pneumonia in ambulatory children 3 to 12 years old may be caused by *Mycoplasma pneumoniae* or *Chlamydia pneumoniae*, and although *M pneumoniae* is not a pathogen in AOM, *C pneumoniae* is present in up to 8% of cases.

β-Lactam and sulfonamide antibiotics have minimal *in vitro* activity against *M pneumoniae* and *C pneumoniae*, so they would not be a suitable choice. The macrolide antibiotics (azithromycin and clarithromycin) would be the preferred choice because they have shown efficacy for both "atypical" pneumonia pathogens and "typical" AOM pathogens. Erythromycin-sulfisoxazole has a marginal spectrum of *in vitro* efficacy for AOM pathogens, but its effectiveness is limited because of its poor penetration into middle ear effusion (MEE), its dosing regimen (4 times a day), its tendency to cause gastritis, its potential for sulfa drug reaction, and its lack of coverage for *Haemophilus influenzae*.

■ Case 2: Immunized Child Develops High Fever and Moderate Leukocytosis While Receiving Amoxicillin for Persistent AOM

A 15-month-old child, who is fully immunized, becomes moderately ill while receiving standard-dose amoxicillin (40 mg/kg divided tid) for treatment of persistent AOM. He has high fever and moderate leukocytosis and his lungs are clear and no sign of meningitis is present. The *H influenzae* type B vaccine has virtually eliminated infections caused by *H influenzae* type B. The use of pneumococcal conjugate vaccine (PCV)–7 (Prevnar) use has also markedly reduced invasive disease caused by penicillin-nonsusceptible *Streptococcus pneumoniae* (PNSP), however, PNSP is still a possibility. Thus in this child with disease refractory to amoxicillin, bacteremia or early pneumonia due to PNSP is most likely. Hospitalization may be necessary but outpatient therapy may be an option if the child is not severely ill, if caregivers seem trustworthy to administer medication and monitor the child's health, and if very close follow-up is possible for the first 24 hours. If outpatient therapy is planned, blood cultures should be obtained to rule out bacteremia. Lack of improvement requires a chest radiograph and hospitalization.

If the child has not been fully immunized with PCV-7 and symptoms are severe or include the gastrointestinal (GI) tract, the first choice for therapy is ceftriaxone (50 mg/kg/d) administered intramuscularly daily for 3 days. The success rate for treatment of PNSP in AOM with ceftriaxone is high, but the effectiveness of therapy should be carefully monitored for the first 24 to 48 hours.

■ Case 3: Bilateral Purulent Conjunctivitis With AOM

A 10-month-old patient with AOM refractory to treatment with amoxicillin develops abrupt onset of bilateral purulent conjunctivitis. Up to two thirds of children with purulent conjunctivitis have concurrent AOM. The usual pathogen in conjunctivitis-otitis syndrome is *H influenzae*, and in one population studied recently, 69% of *H influenzae* strains produced β-lactamase. However, *S pneumoniae*, either penicillin-susceptible or PNSP, is occasionally isolated. If Gram's stain or culture results from the eye are negative or not available, appropriate antibiotic selections are amoxicillin-clavulanate or a third-generation cephalosporin (preferably cefdinir, cefixime, or cefpodoxime). Amoxicillin would not be a first-line choice.

Trimethoprim/sulfamethoxazole (TMP/SMX) is also a consideration only in areas where *H influenzae* is reasonably susceptible.

Other cephalosporins are not good choices to treat AOM with conjunctivitis because they have less *in vitro* coverage or efficacy against β-lactamase–producing *H influenzae*. Newer macrolides also would not be ideal because of lesser activity against *H influenzae,* whether β-lactamase–producing or not.

■ **Case 4: Lymphadenitis and Impetigo**
   Develop in Child With AOM

An 18-month-old patient with AOM who has completed 2 days of amoxicillin therapy develops lymphadenitis and impetigo of the nose. Although *Staphylococcus aureus* is a rare cause of AOM, it is cultured in 95% of cases of impetigo and lymphadenitis of bacterial origin. In addition, group A streptococcus, which are cultured alone in 5% of cases of impetigo, should have responded to amoxicillin. Thus this patient is infected with at least two pathogens: *S aureus* and the usual pathogen(s) causing AOM. Nearly all strains of *S aureus* produce β-lactamase, rendering amoxicillin ineffective.

Up to 20% of *S aureus* isolates are resistant to macrolide antibiotics and resistance to cefaclor is increasingly being reported, so these medications are not the first choice in this patient. Cefdinir is the only third-generation cephalosporin with more than minimal efficacy against *S aureus* at recommended pediatric dosages, although cefpodoxime is approved at double the standard dose only in adults. The second-generation cephalosporin cefuroxime axetil has shown good efficacy against *S aureus*, although it is the least palatable of the oral antibiotic agents for AOM. Cefprozil could also be considered in this scenario. TMP-SMX also has reasonable efficacy against *S aureus* but no activity against PNSP and marginal activity against *H influenzae*. Therefore, preferred antibiotics to treat impetigo due to *S aureus* and AOM due to an unknown pathogen in this patient would be amoxicillin-clavulanate, cefdinir, or cefprozil.

■ Case 5: Persistent Vomiting and Diarrhea Develop in Patient With AOM During Amoxicillin Treatment

A 30-month-old child who has been receiving amoxicillin for 9 days has developed persistent vomiting and diarrhea and is found to have bulging, erythematous tympanic membranes (TMs). The choice of second-line therapy for this child with GI disturbance and AOM due to penicillin-resistant pathogen(s) should be based on minimizing GI tract effects (eliminating amoxicillin-clavulanate, clarithromycin, and erythromycin-sulfisoxazole) and optimizing palatability (eliminating cefuroxime, clarithromycin, and cefpodoxime). The only antibiotics with better *in vitro* efficacy against both PNSP and β-lactamase–producing *H influenzae* with milder GI side effects and better palatability are cefdinir and possibly azithromycin. However, azithromycin should be avoided if bacterial enteritis is suspected (high fever or blood or leukocytes in the stool), because it lacks good coverage for enteric pathogens and has poor serum concentration. Cefixime has minimal PNSP coverage. This is an ideal patient for tympanocentesis if it is available.

■ Case 6: AOM Persists During Azithromycin Treatment In a Fully Vaccinated Child

An 18-month-old male patient who has received his fourth dose of PCV-7 presents to the office with irritability, nighttime restlessness, and ear tugging. He has just completed a course of azithromycin prescribed in the emergency department for a previous initial episode of AOM. His TMs are still full and opacified with a purulent effusion. He is afebrile, previously healthy, and has no medication allergies.

According to data from Dagan and colleagues comparing amoxicillin-clavulanate with azithromycin for AOM, the suspected most likely causative pathogen would be *H influenzae*. A smaller percentage of cases would be accounted for by PNSP, particularly in light of data from Eskola and associates. Their data on AOM in Finnish children showed that PCV-7's coverage of vaccine-serotype–specific strains of *S pneumoniae* (regardless of penicillin susceptibility) in AOM was 57%. Subsequently, a fully vaccinated child should have moderate protection in AOM against the five serotypes that usually account for most PNSP strains. Thus preferred antibiotic choices would be amoxicillin/clavulanate, cefdinir, or cefpodoxime, all of which possess good activity against *H influenzae* and reasonable activity against PNSP.

SUGGESTED READING

Block SL. Strategies for dealing with amoxicillin failure in acute otitis media. *Arch Fam Med.* 1999;8:68-78.

Block SL, Hedrick J, Harrison CJ, et al. Pneumococcal serotypes from acute otitis media in rural Kentucky. *Pediatr Infect Dis J.* 2002;21:859-865.

Block SL, Hedrick J, Tyler R, et al. Increasing bacterial resistance in pediatric acute conjunctivitis (1997-1998). *Antimicrob Agents Chemother.* 2000;44:1650-1654.

Dagan R, Johnson CE, McLinn S, et al. Bacteriologic and clinical efficacy of amoxicillin/clavulanate vs azithromycin in acute otitis media. *Pediatr Infect Dis J.* 2000;19:95-104.

Eskola J, Kilpi T, Palmu A, et al. Efficacy of a pneumococcal conjugate vaccine against acute otitis media. *N Engl J Med.* 2001;344:403-409.

INDEX

Note: Entries followed by "f" indicate figures; "t" indicate tables.

13

13

13

13

13

13

13

13

13

13

13

13